The MIND Method

Re-wiring the Brain to Overcome ADHD, Dyslexia, Autism, Anxiety, Seizures, TBI, and Other Neuro-Behavioral Disorders

Dr. Russ Schroder

Functional Neurologist

and Dr. Heather Schroder

Doctor of Naturopathy

Director: Neuro Care/ MIND Institute for Neurological Development

While the authors have made every effort to provide accurate resources (Internet addresses, etc.) at the time of this publication, we assume no responsibility for errors or for changes that occur post-publication. Further, the authors have no control over nor assume responsibility for any third-party websites or their content.

The authors do not diagnose, treat, cure, or prevent any disease or medical conditions, nor offer medical advice pertaining to treatment or medication usage. Statements contained within have not been approved by the FDA, but if the FDA wanted to be free of bias in the first place, then they should stop receiving millions of dollars in funding from the drug companies.

Thoughts and ideas contained within are strictly informational and not meant to diagnose, treat, cure, or prevent any disease. You are advised to consult with a health care professional with regards to matters relating to your health and in particular regarding matters that may require diagnosis or medical attention.

ISBN-13: 978-1495244995

ISBN-10: 1495244997

Cover design by Tony Rose
Illustrations by Russel Schroder

ALSO BY DR. RUSS SCHRODER

BUCKET LIST: AVENGERS!
A FUNCTIONAL NEUROLOGIST'S EXTRA EXPERIENCE IN THE #3 MOVIE
OF ALL-TIME!

DEDICATIONS

R.S.

This book is dedicated to Heather and "the girls," Riley and Marlee.
To my Mom and Dad. Every day I try to live up to the standards you
set for me. I want to make you proud.
To the eminent neuroscientist, Dr. Frederick "Ted" Carrick for his
wisdom and his dedication to alleviating the suffering of humanity.
As the "Grandfather of Functional Neurology," his energy hasn't
faded as he continually strives to help ease the suffering of mankind.
To Dr. Robert Melillo who has carried on and expanded Dr.
Carrick's work. Thank you for the guidance.
To Dr. Jinaan Jawad for pushing me.
To Dr. Dan Murphy who taught me the word Paleo.
And to Dr. Jeremy Martin for introducing me to Neurofeedback.
Also, this book is dedicated to our clients.

H.S.

These stories couldn't have happened without the amazing families
we've had the privilege to work with during this journey. You have
all made our dream a reality.

Thank you to my parents for making me a fighter throughout all the
ups and downs of my unhealthy → healthy life. You've taught me to
seek answers, to improve my life, instead of accepting it as a death
sentence or a loss. You never let me get down or feel sorry for
myself. I have never given up during those hard times and it's thanks
to the "fighter attitude" you've instilled in me.

To my daughters, Riley and Marlee. You are my everything. You helped me discover the joy of children. I hope to be as good of a role model to you as you are to me. Seeing you struggle and grow developmentally and academically has pushed me to learn more so I can give you the best life possible.

And none of these "Thank you's" would be possible without ever knowing Dr. Russ. Our passion for neurology has brought us together personally and professionally. You've helped free me from my "death sentence." You believed in my crazy ideas and even helped them to become a reality.

The MIND Method and MIND Institute would not be in existence without the support of all these wonderful people.

Thank you all!

Heather and Dr. Russ would *both* like to thank Dr. Connie Schroder and Sharon Williams for proof-reading original drafts of this book… and for just being great moms.

CONTENTS

FOREWORD

It is a powerful statement to *you*, the reader, that you are sitting down in front of this piece of work. It means that you care enough about your (or a loved one's) health to take the time to learn what science knows about the brain as of 2014.

Heather and Dr. Russ have taken some very complicated, well-referenced material and broken it down in a simplified manner so you can understand the benefits and consequences of living in the modern world. It's a marvelous time to be alive. That's for sure!

We have the greatest technology and access to the greatest information known to mankind. The internet was originally designed for researchers at universities to share data-sets, after all. And now it is at our finger-tips!

However, our environment isn't what it used to be. The "fish full of mercury" that Marvin Gaye warned us about in 1971 have only gotten worse. Our food supply is tainted with pesticides that contribute to Leaky Gut Syndrome (or "intestinal permeability" if you want to research its technical, scientific name).

Our cows, chicken, fish and pigs are being fed corn against their biological needs (against their genetics), causing inflammatory chemicals to be absorbed through *our* gut walls into our cells and nerves.

Our school systems are having increasing difficulties managing the incredibly high volume of children with neurobehavioral disorders. Our elderly are getting dementias and Alzheimer's at rapidly rising rates! It is a growing national emergency!

It has been a pleasure to get to know Dr. Russ and Heather over the past few years. Every time we sit down for dinner after a conference, they are updating me about the need to constantly stay on the cutting edge of science and nutrition.

In a nutshell, their 3 pronged approach at the MIND Institute for Neurological Development (The MIND Method) is Neurofeedback, Neurology and Nutrition.

It is simply stunning with the care and speed at which they are able to change peoples' lives for the better. Dr. Russ introduced me to Cold Laser and Neurofeedback at a Neurology conference a while back and I am still amazed with the results!

Most importantly, I hope that *you* will be, too. That's really the joy of being a doctor. It's helping patients in need. It's giving Quality of Life back. It's the smiles and "thank you's" that you get when you are doing your job… and doing it well!

My hope is that you finish this book and keep it handy for future reference. It's about the future of our planet. It's about the future of our children.

May you get everything that you need out of this book, and more importantly, out of life.

Dr. Jinaan Jawad

Functional Neurologist

INTRODUCTION

"Who are you going to believe, me or you own eyes?"
– Groucho Marx

Today, as you are reading this, over one thousand *more* Americans are diagnosed with a condition involving abnormal function of the human brain.

Each year, 13-20 percent of children living in the USA experience some form of mental disorder, and the prevalence is on the rise. (CDC- Centers for Disease Control and Prevention, Six County Inc.)

ADHD/ADD was the most commonly reported with behavioral problems, anxiety, depression and autism following behind.

ADHD and Autism are at all time highs with 1 in 10 children diagnosed with Attention Deficit/Hyperactivity Disorder. While Autism is found in *at least* 1 in 88 children. (2013 stats say 1 in 50!)

Clinical Depression and Anxiety in the U.S. is estimated at 1 in 5 people.

Millions of adults and youths *as young as 4* play contact sports such as football, hockey, soccer and lacrosse resulting in hundreds of concussions (or mTBI- "mild" Traumatic Brain Injury) each and every single day.

Add to that the soldiers returning from at least 2 conflicts (more accurately: "Wars") who are saved by protective gear that prevents death but cannot prevent damage from the concussive forces *inside* the human skull, leaving their brains cooking in inflammation, shattering their lives, ruining their relationships.

Over a million kids in school right now have difficulty reading due to transposing letters, seeing words "backwords" or letters upside down or backwards. (Dyslexia)

Seizure disorders and epilepsy are also rising at an unprecedented rate with no end in sight. These patients' brains are so unstable that they can't even maintain the basic homeostatic baseline to function, over-firing when not squashed by inhibitory medications.

In Muskingum County alone, Six County Inc. saw an increase in youth with mental problems from 323 in 2008 to *1,196* in 2012! That's a nearly *400% INCREASE* in just the past 4 years.

The 3 most common were ADHD, anxiety and depression. (Times Recorder 11/10/13)

In Anatomy of An Epidemic, Robert Whitaker correctly points out that when the final analysis is done, pharmaceutical medications are being sought out as the treatment of choice in many cases due to their ease of use, *despite* the fact that overwhelming evidence points directly to the conclusion that the cure IS worse than the disease. We are now at the point in human history where the medications we take are causing even worse problems than the primary reason we started them in the first place.

It is with the hope of helping an entire population from becoming "Generation Rx" that we present this book to you.

- The Authors

1. A TROUBLED BRAIN - HEATHER'S STORY

"The greatest thing, then, is to make our nervous system our ally instead of our enemy."
– William James, 19th Century American Philosopher

My story: by Heather Bennett (now Heather Schroder, ND)

PART 1 – MY CHILDHOOD

I've always been a complicated case. My family physician referred to me as a "top priority patient." Being sick was all I ever really knew. I always had *some* bizarre illness.

My mom got pregnant for me when she was 14 years old but didn't even know it. She always had irregular periods and no one talked to her about sex or it's consequences.

Mom had some weight gain, so she was seen by her family doctor. Because of her age and always being sick herself, no one thought to run a pregnancy test. Instead, it was "determined" that she had an overactive thyroid and was placed on thyroid medication.

She later found out that she was actually *pregnant* when my aunt bumped her belly, feeling me kick! By the time my mother got to the doctor, almost six months had passed. Because of the lack of prenatal care, I was born almost a month early!

The health issues started at birth. Due to jaundice, I was placed in an incubator for a few days. (My baby picture looks like an alien!... No hair. No eyebrows. No eyelashes or fingernails. It would be 3 decades later after a rare medication reaction that these would all fall off again!) My facial features also weren't very prominent.

Growing up I had many ear infections. In kindergarten and first grade I was in speech therapy for talking too fast and not being able to pronounce my O's, R's, or L's. I even had a lazy eye which really became prominent when I was tired.

I believe it was in the first grade when I had my first "passing out" spell.

We were all lined up in the gym to receive a vaccination, I'm not even sure what kind it was, but my memory is that of a sci-fi gun that spun to the next round after each shot. The class was lined up to go back to the room. I remember looking at the back of the line, when the next thing I know I was on the ground with several teachers standing over me!

That's pretty much all I remember. (A seizure at age 20 took much of my early memories). The next few years were typical childhood issues, thankfully! Chicken pox, the flu, a broken ankle. I was happy and healthy with lots of friends. And I was very active.

Fourth grade was the turning point for my health, again. Two months before my 10th birthday, I had my first seizure.

It was a Sunday morning. My mom and I were getting ready for Sunday school. She remembers curling my bangs and yelling at me to hold still because I was fidgeting, when all of a sudden she realized I was "staring right through her!"

So she shook me to bring me out of it, but I fell backwards, hitting my head on a vanity drawer. She said I was as stiff as a board with my eyes rolled back in my head!

She ran to get my dad who carried me to the kitchen. While she was on the phone calling an ambulance, I regained my consciousness. I was screaming at the top of my lungs and crying.

I slept the entire rest of the day.

I had my first EEG (Electro-encephalogram) shortly after. The results showed abnormal brain activity. Combined with an asymmetrical CT ("cat") scan showing one side of my brain was bigger than the other, I was diagnosed with a seizure disorder.

The seizures hadn't occurred for several years, but I had begun to notice other changes. I started having trouble in school (besides fainting). Prior to the seizure, I was at the top in math class. There was even talk of me moving up a grade. Post-seizure, my concentration and comprehension was just horrible. I had to be put in the second to lowest math group.

This was a huge blow to my delicate self-esteem already. I began having emotional issues. My feelings were being hurt more often. I was angry. I felt like an outcast. I felt different. I just didn't know what was wrong with me.

Around 5th or 6th grade, I started hyperventilating. There really were no triggers. My mother bought me bright yellow lunch bags with smiley faces on them as my special bags to breathe into.

In 7th grade, I began having "staring spells" in class. (These were likely Absence seizures that went undiagnosed). At a parent teacher conference, my mom was told that I day-dreamed a lot. Neither had thought of seizures because I didn't lose consciousness or convulse.

But I recall coming out of these spells (which I call "black out spells") not remembering what was just said in class. I was falling behind, but because I was so shy, I was afraid to ask for help!

PART 2 – MY TEEN YEARS

At age 15, I had 2 episodes in the same morning while getting ready for school. I don't even remember the details.

But once I was taken to our family doctor, it was determined that I had a seizure followed by a slight stroke. The doctor ordered an MRI.

It was a difficult wait. A few days later my mom received a phone call saying the MRI showed a "spot" on my brain the size of a pencil eraser (on the inner cerebrum). It was labeled a tumor. However, due to the location, a biopsy was not recommended in order to prevent nerve damage.

For the next year, I had numerous MRI's to monitor my brain: from weekly for a month, to bi-weekly, to monthly to bi-monthly to finally every six months. Fortunately, the tumor disappeared on its own without treatment.

Throughout high school, I had issues with feeling over-heated. I couldn't be outside for very long or I was likely to pass out. It wasn't really seizure activity. (I was already put on medication for an irregular heartbeat my 8th grade year).

I experienced burning sensations in the back of my head whenever I turned it. I called it "fizzing" since it felt like something was popping followed by "fizzing" in my neck up into my skull. There was no real explanation for this, but I was given cortisone shots where the base of my skull meets the top of my neck. I received these injections every six months for two years! (But it never helped ease the popping or fizzing).

After graduating high school, I started college, worked a part time job and got married (pretty much what a typical American girl would do, but all at once!)

Soon, the black out spells began again. In fact, I had 10 to 20 *per day!* I tried to dismiss them. They would happen like flipping off a light switch. Sudden. Unexpected. Often they would jolt me when I came back around.

They became even more frequent, more intense. Soon, I was even having seizures in which I was losing bladder function. My parents took me to consult with a new neurologist.

He prescribed Calan for mini-strokes. But to no avail. I had episodes where I woke up with horrible stomach cramps and a bowel movement so aggressive that it felt like a near-death experience!

I described it as the "Alice in Wonderland" effect. (Neurologists say patients will feel small in a big world or big in a small world, or like they're falling- each of which occurs in the story when Alice goes down the rabbit hole). These are also associated with Geshwind syndrome, both by-products of Temporal lobe epilepsy ("repetitive seizures emanating from the temporal lobe").

I would also break out in a cold sweat, with a dry mouth and racing heart. I would pass out and then wake myself from it squealing in a high pitch. I would try to get up but my body was so limp. My bowels would release all over me while lying face down on the floor.

After the second time of this happening, my husband eventually left and filed for divorce.

None of the doctors on hand had any kind of explanation for this. One doctor said it was an allergic reaction to milk.

PART 3- MY 20'S

About six months later I had my worst seizure ever. I came home from work and had been battling a migraine all day. I was living back at home with my parents, having had my drivers licensed revoked for medical purposes. (They didn't want me to seize while driving on the road).

One night, my mom and I had ordered a pizza. I remember eating a mushroom, and that's it. That's all I can remember from that day. My mom told me she was sitting with me in the kitchen when I fell over backwards, my body seizing up "like an accordion," my hands clawing at the floor, my face clenched in agony.

We lived next to the ambulance station, so when she called they were there in minutes. Timing it at just under 10 minutes, by the time the squad had arrived, I did not have a pulse nor was I breathing, but I was STILL seizing! After an EMT put a tube up my nose, I finally came out of it.

I was transported to the ER where I was given a horrendous cocktail of 1000 mg of Tylenol, 1000 mg of Tegretol (an "anti-seizure" medication), 1000 mg of Dilantin, and 1000 mg of Phenobarbitol. I was coherent but having hallucinations from all the meds.

The clock on the wall looked like it was melting (like in a Salvador Dali painting). It felt like an army of ants was crawling all over me and down the bed. I later described the kids in the hallway as "midget wrestlers" (costumes and all).

My mother had to get me down to the car by herself when I was released. By 15, I was taller than her. Now, here I am, at 20 and using her as a crutch just to make it home. She said I never woke up all day Saturday.

She tried to wake me to get me to eat, but as she started to prop me up but my head would start bobbing as I had no muscle control throughout my entire body. One of the EMT's was even nice enough to stop by to check on me. After seeing my condition, he urged my parents to take me back to the hospital for further treatment. So, my mother called the nurse-line for confirmation. They said to give me fluids and keep me hydrated. But every time I tried to drink, I started seizing again. So they got me into the car right away.

While driving me there, a deep wave of concern washed over them. I was talking out of my head. Absolute nonsense. I wanted my cat. My childhood toys. Coloring books and crayons. My ex-husband. And other bizarre rants.

The doctor on duty ordered a spinal tap. He advised my parents to hold me in the fetal position since it is such a painful procedure.

I slept through the entire procedure... Without moving... A SPINAL TAP!

The doctor drew a vial of clear fluid from my spine. He said he had never seen anything like it. He had only read about it in the textbooks. Too much fluid in the spinal canal could put pressure on the brain.

Prior to the tap I had told my parents that I thought we were at the circus because the I.V. hooks and bags looked like cotton candy. Seconds later my parents said I thought that *they* were the doctors and I was screaming at them not to touch me!

I was admitted to the hospital for 5 days (the ICU for 1 of them). The first couple days, I was basically in a coma. When I came out of it, I can honestly say that was a turning point in my "New Life."

My uncle Jamie and I were always close, but when he came to visit me, I didn't know who he was! There were several other close friends and family members who also visited me that I didn't remember either!

I had trouble walking. My body looked mangled. My feet and hands were curled inwards. Whenever I tried to get out of bed, I fell to the floor.

My family "doctor" told my parents that I had "faked the whole thing for attention" because of the recent divorce. He actually argued this belief with my neurologist, in front of my parents! The neurologist had to explain that due to the severity of the seizure and the intense muscle spasms that resulted, it would be *impossible* for me to walk!

That was the last time I saw my family doctor.

After a decade of having seizures, I was finally diagnosed with epilepsy and prescribed a daily dose of Tegretol (to reduce brain activity and therefore reduce the epileptic spikes of brain over-firing).

When I got home from the hospital, my family and I had to make a lot of changes. I had to learn how to do my hair and make-up again (and I used to do runway modeling in high-school! I used to do my hair and make-up almost every day before all this happened). I had exercises I had to do to learn to walk again.

My personality even changed. I went from being angry, even hostile, to a kinder, gentler person. Calmer.

Yet, ever since that seizure, I've had trouble remembering many events from childhood to high school. My short term memory-loss had kicked into high gear. I couldn't remember what was just said to me and I began having issues with repeating myself frequently.

Staying positive and refusing to give up, I started college. It allowed me the chance to focus on my passion, kids. While I was learning the ropes, working up to my degree in Early Childhood Development, I met my first child with autism.

I was so drawn to him. I'd work 1-on-1 with him as often as I could, observing his movements, looking for the rationale for his behavior. I quickly became a magnet to the difficult children, the ones no one else thought were fun. I felt that since my childhood was misunderstood due to my "disabilities," I was meant to make a life helping those children.

My first year teaching was certainly a challenge. I felt this was me being thrown into the deep end to sink or swim. I had several ADHD children, kids with speech impediments (like I once had), fetal alcohol syndrome, and another autistic child who was legally blind and hearing impaired.

When I switched schools, the typical kids weren't as much of a passion. The occasional ADHD and bipolar ones really tugged at my heart. (One bipolar child had been diagnosed at age 3!) I wanted so badly to take these kids home with me. Although, they were labeled as "bad," I found they were quite loveable with hearts of gold.

After years of being able to identify kids with disabilities, I once told a parent their 3 year-old was likely autistic. He had lots of solitary play, poor motor coordination, delayed speech, hand flapping and rocking. His head was also enlarged. The mother agreed to speech and OT/PT (occupational and physical therapy) services but was denied care because he was "too young to know for sure." I ran into her a few years later, and sure enough, at age 7, he was finally diagnosed with Autism.

(The years of teaching dance taught me to identify children with poor motor coordination. It has become a blessing and a curse to observe children in public, seeing poor rhythms, balance and cross-body movements associated with weaknesses in the brain, knowing what I know now, that many children are unfairly diagnosed with Dyslexia, ADHD or other neuro-behavioral disabilities that could benefit from what is now being called *brain-based* care).

It was during this time teaching that I was able to finally get my Driver's license back. I was actually doing well with the Tegretol.

And two years after that, I was re-married and even pregnant! This, despite the fact that several doctors had told me that I would never be able to get pregnant because of a tilted uterus.

I was at work one day and had the "Alice in Wonderland" effect. This didn't seem right considering the dosage of Tegretol I was on. So, on a hunch, I went home after a short stop at a pharmacy and took a pregnancy test… And then two more…

They were all positive.

My neurologist had released me to the care of my *new* family doctor because the seizures were otherwise controlled. So, they kept me on the current dose of Tegretol, as prevention, while I was carrying my first daughter, Riley. I made it through the pregnancy without any seizures, but after she was born, (bald but beautiful!) Riley had "breath-holding spells" that the doctors thought might have been a side-effect or signs of her being "addicted" to the meds I took.

When I found out two years later that I was pregnant for my second daughter, Marlee (also beautiful and bald!), the new family doctor felt I was doing well enough that I could be taken off the meds in order to have a healthy pregnancy. I actually had no seizures and no issues with her!

After she was born, my seizures quickly returned. And different ones this time. An all new breed, if you will. These were a "whole 'nother animal." So, back on the Tegretol.

Whenever I would stand up from a seated or lying position, I'd pass out. Just lights out. Crumple to the floor. Then wake up a few seconds to a minute later.

I was fine just sitting down and relaxing. Except that I would still have some "Alice in Wonderland's" kick in, and the migraines were back.

PART 4 – MY 30'S

My marriage was in trouble. My husband couldn't handle me being sick all the time. He either ignored me or got mad when I was having a seizure. Several times he would slap me in the face while I was seizing. As a certified CPR and First-Aid instructor, he believed dragging his knuckles across my sternum was proper care of a seizing patient. One time he dumped a cup full of ice water in my face.

Often times he said I faked it.

I eventually went back to my neurologist who referred me to a cardiologist. He performed an echo-cardiogram and stress test. That's when they determined I had low sodium. So, unlike 98% of America, I would need to *add* salt to my diet daily. Beef jerky became my go-to food.

I lost my driving privileges again, this time for a month. The seizures continued but not as bad around this time.

Once I knew the trigger, I began to notice the effect of low sodium on my body. My right eye would twitch… literally the eye… The muscles that move the eyeball. Not the muscles of the face that blink or open the eye. My eyeball would twitch!

My face would go numb, too. Once I had my "sodium fix" though, my symptoms would usually dissipate. Other times, the numbness would travel to the left side of my face. When this happened, I would crash and go into a full blown seizure.

After that, whenever I would "feel a seizure coming on," (Neurologists call this the "aura"- "symptoms that herald the onset of a seizure" – Netter's Neurology 2007) I would try to fight it as long as I could to get to a safe place. Yes, safety from the seizures, but also from my husband.

In 2007, I left teaching to start a dance studio for two years. During those years I drank a LOT of Mountain Dew. 10-12 cans per day! And interestingly enough, I had very *very* few seizures. I was also constantly moving. What an amazing feeling. I was so energetic and happy!

The Tegretol was leaving me feeling sluggish and numb when I took it. So, I was switched to Lamictal in October of that year. I immediately felt a difference. I actually didn't even feel medicated for the first time in 10 years!

PART 5 – "SJS"

Nothing this good could last. A week after starting the Lamictal, I noticed some other changes as well. The lymph nodes in my neck were protruding. In my mind, I thought I looked like Frankenstein's monster. The doctor at Urgent Care believed I had a viral infection. "Fair enough," I thought "My girls had been sick."

By the 10th day on the new drug, after finding and reading the warning label brochure, I saw my symptoms next to the letters "SJS" in *red* letters. I knew that I was having an allergic reaction. It was a Friday morning and by noon a rash appeared on my belly. By 8 that evening, the rash had spread all over and my throat was swelling up!

My husband was playing poker and always kept his phone off. For whatever reason I couldn't reach my parents either. So I dropped my daughters off at their other grandmother's house to spend the evening in the Emergency Room. The doctor on duty that night diagnosed it as a viral infection, gave me an anaphylactic shot, then released me.

I stayed with my parents that night. The next morning I was in misery. Even the whites of my eyes were red as the rash had now spread to my *entire* body! It felt like a million little bees stinging me repeatedly. My tongue was swollen- making it hard to swallow. My lips were so big. They felt flipped inside out! (My dad even said they looked bigger than Angelina Jolie's lips... not something I ever wanted).

I tried to call my family doctor to no avail. He was out of town. Sure enough, his replacement sent me to the E.R. Again, more shots and "viral infection" diagnosis.

Sunday my mom stayed with me. I took scalding hot baths several times to help numb the pain. I packed oatmeal paste on the rash. I knew scratching would cause scars, so I slapped myself when the itching got unbearable.

Mom's hamburger helper felt like tiny   rocks in my mouth. Thrush was forming in my mouth by this time. My tongue was turning grey. E.R. again. Shots and same diagnosis. On the way home I passed out, which meant my mom had to fireman's carry me in. My husband just stood there and watched.

Around 3 A.M. Monday morning, I was wheezing, feeling tightness in my chest, and having difficulty breathing. I was gasping for air, begging my husband to take me back to the ER. Instead, he called 911. In the squad I was given yet *another* anaphylactic shot.

I had a seizure and don't remember a thing about the visit.

At the E.R., I was given- you guessed it- same diagnosis, same shots, with prednisone as a kicker. On the way home, my mother said she had to steer with her left hand and hold my head with her right hand because I began seizing yet *again*. She had to fireman's carry me, *again*, into my house after my husband gave up trying to pull my stiff, contracted, seized-up body out of the passenger seat. They said I barely even moaned throughout the whole process!

Later that morning I called my neurologist and explained what was going on. He said to stop the Lamictal immediately because I was having an allergic reaction. (This was no surprise. I had already stopped it on Saturday because of the warning label.) He declined to see me before my scheduled appointment on Wednesday, though. Frustrated, I called my family doctor for advice (besides just stopping the reaction-inducing medication and pretending I had a viral infection that the ER docs so desperately wanted me to have).

He wanted to see me right away. This was the week of Thanksgiving in Ohio. Typical cold, seasonal weather, but I was wearing flip-flops, shorts and a tank top. No bra. I was in such misery. My nervous system was being so damaged that I couldn't tell if it was hot or cold.

The doctor examined me and gave me a one in a million diagnosis. Stevens-Johnson Syndrome. "SJS." A very rare reaction to medications. Being diagnosed with it is like winning the lottery.

Only the pay-outs are some of the strangest symptoms ever. Cell death causes the skin's dermis and epidermis layers to separate!

I had ulcers from the inside to the outside of my body. I had such a severe yeast infection that the infection was green. I was so weak that I just didn't care what was being done to me. He admitted me to the hospital immediately.

As soon as I got there, a dermatologist met me with a team of *six* doctors! They had medical books, clip-boards and cameras. I was a textbook case- never seen by anyone in our area before! My gown was lifted as the doctors took measurements and photos of the ulcers. They asked me so may questions about my medical past. They confirmed my doctor's initial diagnosis of SJS with a crossover of "TEN"/ Toxic Epidermal Necrolysis- both life-threatening!

One of the medical staff even said I should have been transported to Columbus' Riverside Hospital to the burn-victims unit because the team in Zanesville didn't really know how to care for me properly. (I was given so much medication that I didn't even know what I had. I just slept my whole week there.)

On Tuesday, my second night in the hospital, my aunt was visiting me when the heart monitor began beeping erratically. When the nurses came running in, they informed her I was going into cardiac arrest! Thankfully, I was stabilized quickly, but it was quite a shock to be told this later by my concerned aunt.

I knew my heart was skipping beats, but not enough to consider it a major deal. Then the unlucky lottery symptoms began.

My hair fell out. On the back of my head at first. Then it moved forward.

Then my eyebrows and lashes began falling out.

Then my fingernails started coming loose. Then they fell off.

I woke up one morning as the skin from my lips sloughed off onto my pillow. I couldn't shave because my blood wouldn't clot. (Plus, I worried I would shave my skin off!)

The Thanksgiving meal at the hospital was disgusting. I think. I mean I couldn't actually taste it. But the texture felt awful. It tasted salty even though it was sodium-free.

I was released a week after being admitted. The releasing doctor said I might be a good candidate for a *brain implant* that fires electrical charges to disrupt seizures as they begin. "That's re-assuring" I thought, not sure if I meant it or was secretly being sarcastic with myself.

In an effort to get back to my life without dwelling on what had just happened, I went immediately back to teaching at the dance studio. The next two months of recovery were tough on me.

It was the dead of winter, but here I am still in flip-flops and t-shirts. No coat. Because my nervous system, immune system, and soft tissues were so compromised, I still couldn't tell if I was hot or cold. Or hungry. Or full.

I went grocery shopping during that first week out and bumped my head on the hatch unloading bags. I knew I bumped it. I heard it. And felt my head stop suddenly. I just didn't know I'd hit it hard enough to gush blood.

When I ate, I kept eating until the food was gone. I was never satiated. Every time I went to the kitchen, I got a drink because I didn't know if I was thirsty or not. Water and milk became the only two beverages I'd drink, but I couldn't even taste a difference. (My old favorite, Mountain Dew, tasted like flat, green popsicles. Disgusting).

Going to the bathroom was difficult since I no longer felt the sensory input telling me if my bowel or bladder was full.

Sleeping was next to impossible. The ulcers were healing, scaling, and sticking to my clothes and bed linens. At night, I would sweat out the toxins. It smelled like burnt flesh. Coughing fits would produce white dry particles. I was later informed that this was my esophagus' lining coming up.

The first week back at the dance studio was hard. I would go through bursts of immense energy to feeling completely drained a half hour later. I couldn't feel the floor under my feet nor could I point my toes. One of my students never returned after grabbing me by the hands and accidentally pulling off a fingernail.

The thrush was so bad, I had to see my dentist because my teeth were loosening. Week 2, I visited my eye doctor due to all the trouble with my eyes. He said that because of the soft tissue and immune system damage, I wasn't able to produce tears! I was advised to have corneal replacements as the dryness often caused my lid to stick to my cornea when I would blink!

Despite all this, I was slowly starting to recover. Then, about 2 months later I had a setback, when some seafood caused a breakout. An ingredient found in shellfish *and* in the Lamictal drug caused another allergic reaction.

They put me on steroids for about three months. The combination of health issues, marriage issues, and medication reactions made me very depressed. I tanned daily for that year to help with the scars. (both physical and mental- the tanning produced vitamin D in my skin and helped my moods. I know now how and why it can be addictive).

But again, my husband wasn't able to handle the seizures. Once, he even dug his knuckles into my breast-bone so hard, it resulted in a bruised sternum.

A year later, throughout 2008, I had gained 40 pounds. To keep my spirit up, I would joke that the best part of SJS was going from a B cup to a DD cup!

I gave up the dance studio and started a new job in social work. My first cases were at-risk infants and toddlers. I worked with families, many teen mothers and even developmentally challenged parents on how to appropriately care for their children, helping them meet their milestones. Long before meeting Dr. Russ, I was into tracking infants eyes, playing games to get them targeting. Until he and I started our long discussions on neurology, I hadn't realized I was performing eye pursuits (slow eye movements) and "saccades" (sudden eye movements).

I was busy teaching parents the importance of babies crawling before walking. Saying no to Johnny-walkers instead of encouraging their use as "free baby-sitters." Telling parents to switch sides when feeding their baby to strengthen the ocular-eye muscles, the neck and stimulating both sides of the brain. I knew these were normal protocols for child development but never the neurological reasons why... until much later.

I switched gears from working with easy-going infants and pre-schoolers to children aged 5 to 17 with mental health issues.

I was amazed (and sickened) by how medications were forced onto families' children "to make them better." It was a tough job, knowing how awful I felt being on the Tegretol. How was I going to "make" these parents give their children medications that could alter their child's brain (have suicidal or homicidal thoughts as side-effects) or make them sick? It was my job to enforce the rules even if it meant reporting families to children services for "medical" neglect!

This job was the experience that opened my eyes to the dominance of the pharmaceutical industry. A 9 year old on 14 different behavioral meds??? How were these children able to develop appropriately? Many sat like zombies staring into space while the parents and teachers usually *liked* the new, compliant little Johnny. (See Chapter 7)

But a 5 year old having suicidal and homicidal thoughts shortly after being placed on Abilify? The cocktail of medications counteracting one another creating more diagnoses and thus, more medication!

NO one ever addressed changing their diet! Still a Mountain Dew drinker at that time, I often challenged my clients to see who could go longer without it. Some kids were even drinking Monster and other energy drinks to the point of being admitted to the hospital for "overdosing!"

The positive and negative experiences in those past careers later helped me to work with the families we see now. I know from experience how challenging the system is when teachers, doctors and counselors promote the use of drugs at the expense of helping the child to re-wire the brain naturally!

While getting all this real-world education on how the system is rigged, new health issues started springing up. Why should I expect any less at this point? I wasn't exactly surprised. This was my genetic luck in life, right? The unlucky health lottery?

This time I was having issues with intra-ductal papillomas in my breast tissue. It resolved relatively quickly on its own. For once a health issue was minor. Finally. My health actually began doing better.

Then my youngest daughter was diagnosed with epilepsy. They told us it was hereditary. We participated in a study to support that argument. Was I going to give all this to my girls? Were they doomed to the same genetic traits as me. Would those genes kick on in her at 6 years old?

Again in denial, my husband said Marlee wasn't epileptic. Instead, I just *wanted* our kids to be sick!

Except that the neurologist didn't agree with my husband's diagnosis. He confirmed she *did* have a seizure disorder and placed her on the Tegretol.

Two years after the SJS horror I went through, crippling pains began affecting my arms. It would start as a burning in my right forearm that travelled up to my shoulder and down to my hand, causing me to drop whatever I was holding. Sometimes the numbness would travel over to my left arm, around my back and into my rib cage. Driving was tough. Rain made it worse.

So, I received my newest diagnosis: "Radiculopathy." I relied heavily on Ibuprofen.

It seemed like my health issues were directly linked to SJS. My body was deteriorating.

In 2010, my husband and I filed for divorce. The seizures and IBS were kicking into high gear. That summer, I had a colonoscopy because of bleeding issues thought to be related to Crohn's disease (which runs in my family).

In 2011, I started having trouble at work. It became increasingly difficult to retain information or even do the paperwork I had been using as a social worker for the past 3 years. After an MRI, my neurologist found I had "hippocampal shrinkage," the region of the brain associated with forming long-term memories was reduced by 20%!

A supervisor suggested I get a second opinion so I could file for employees with handicaps. This would allow them to adjust my paperwork and reduce my case-load. Another option was to just file for disability.

I was fired for improper paperwork in May of 2011 despite repeatedly asking for clarification on what the company wanted. I even offered to take training but was denied. Secretly, I feel they weren't making enough money off my case-load, that I was spending too much time with clients, going to their homes, driving them to doctors visits, and "wasting too much company time" consulting with families about their medical, financial and social issues. (I still have former clients greet me enthusiastically when they see me grocery shopping. They say they've never had another social worker give so much).

I followed up for the second opinion in March, just before being let go at work. The office visit was a disaster. The Cleveland Clinic was able to get me in the next day for a consult, but they didn't tell me to bring my stack of medical records. (They actually *told* me I didn't need to bring them! I assumed because of this that they would request them electronically from the local hospital and my neurologist).

They were never sent.

So here I was, trying to explain my health history (the one you've just read) to a new doctor with NO records, NO file, and NO confidence in what I was explaining to her. Even SHE had barely heard of SJS! She looked at me like I was crazy.

She didn't believe a word I said.

I began to cry. How could she not believe me? I truly felt I was going crazy and that perhaps my husband was right. My father was my ride up to the Cleveland Clinic. He wasn't there for most of the doctors visits throughout my life. He was always on the road. Even he thought they might lock me up, the way the Epileptologist (seizure specialist) was dismissing my life story as *pure fiction!*

"Maybe I *was* faking all my health issues," I thought. So, from March to October I began telling myself "I'm *not* epileptic. I'm healthy and there isn't *anything* wrong with me!"

WRONG!

I started back to college, *again,* this time in massage therapy with the goal of being hired on at Children's hospital in Columbus. I could picture myself working with kids again. Working on children with cancer or other debilitating diseases.

To pay for school, I worked part-time as an assistant manager of a retail clothing store. Meanwhile I was driving over an hour to school. All this while being a single mother.

At this time, the seizures started back. This time they were TEN or more in a DAY! Mostly first thing in the morning. I began "passing out" just about every time I stood up. I thought I was tired and overworked.

I would get up at 5 A.M. to get ready and be in Columbus for an 8 o'clock class an hour away. We'd finish up at 3:00, where I would get up cautiously. (I was always trying to hide my passing-out "spells"). Then I would shoot out the door to be at work in Zanesville from 4 until 10 P.M. Afterwards, I'd stay up 'til midnight studying. I was mentally and physically exhausted... but I had *everything* to prove as a single mother of two.

I was living with my parents, sleeping in the cool basement during that summer. I was still trying to convince myself that I wasn't epileptic. I finally caved, calling my neurologist only *after* passing out at the top of the basement stairs. I had slid down every step, resulting in a rug burn that ran from my chin down to the tops of my feet! That and a sprained wrist.

My neurologist did not feel that these new episodes were seizure-related, however. Instead he believed they were coming from an under-lying heart issue.

He sent me to the cardiologist, who ordered me to wear an "event monitor" for the next 30 days. A couple of times the company who monitors the device actually called me because they were receiving readings that were considered at-risk! They told me to report back to the cardiologist immediately. He placed me on sodium and magnesium tablets when this happened.

I was getting ready for work on a Sunday morning when I began to have a sudden pain in my left shoulder that radiated down into my arm. Not surprisingly, the monitoring company called me, urging me to go straight to the ER for a possible heart attack!

After several tests, I was admitted for 3 days. During my stay, they performed a tilt-table test (where you lay on a table and they monitor your heart up-right vs. laying down) and a stress-test where they monitor the heart during exercise. The cardiac results from the tilt-table came back negative even though it caused some of my light-headedness symptoms.

The stress-test was the big shocker. Being physically "fit" (or lean, from dancing most of my life), we were all surprised how in less than a minute I was winded while my eyes became extremely dilated. (A fight-or-flight response). My heart rate went from a resting 60 beats per minute to over 150 b.p.m. in that short time. But my blood pressure *dropped!*

The techs were yelling at me to get off the treadmill immediately before I crashed! I was confused at the urgency. My heart has always felt fast-paced with activity, even though I've always had *low* blood pressure.

A few hours later, the cardiologist on-call came in to tell me (and my parents) that he believed I was misdiagnosed all together. He said that *these* symptoms were from a rare *heart* condition known as P.O.T.S. (Postural Orthostatic Tachycardia Syndrome, simply pronounced as "Pots").

It was explained that because of my low blood pressure, when I would stand up to resume activity after resting, the blood vessels weren't contracting fast enough to aid the heart in *squeezing* the blood up to my brain, so my heart would speed UP, but often times not fast enough to keep enough blood to my brain- causing me to pass out.

His recommendation was a high-sodium diet… and a pacemaker!

He was concerned about inserting a pace-maker, of course. Because of my young age, the number of times they would need to replace it (or the batteries) throughout my lifetime, I would be at risk for infections from surgery every few years!

After being released from the hospital, I had my follow-up appointments with my primary cardiologist and neurologist. The heart doctor agreed with increasing my sodium but balked at implanting a pace-maker in my chest (because of the risk), referring me to an electro-physiologist instead. My neurologist, not wanting to be held liable for any "seizures," refused to remove the "epilepsy" diagnosis. He continued me on Tegretol despite the side-effects.

The electro-physiologist felt my condition was not severe enough... yet. Nor did he feel I was old enough to have a pace-maker. He believed it was only necessary if my condition continued to worsen.

Little did he know, a month later, my life (and health) would change so dramatically!

PART 6 – MEETING DR. RUSS

Working late one night, I was introduced through mutual friends to a man I went to high school with. To put it bluntly, we were set up.

I was told he was a *chiropractor* by my friends and realized that I'd seen his face on a billboard promoting his all-natural program to reverse neuropathy (nerve damage). I guess that I thought he was the hands-on type who adjusts spines all-day, but I learned later that week that while he used to do that, now he does so much more!

He was charming and funny "enough" that I returned his texts later that week, and he asked me about myself. I gave him the "need to know only" facts about my health issues, instead focusing on my time as a teacher, social worker and dance instructor.

That weekend, I got a celebratory text from him stating he passed his *functional* neurology boards. I neither knew he had spent 3 years studying neurology, nor that he was already board certified in chiropractic neurology nor that any other types of neurologists existed except *medical* neurologists.

He politely informed me that neurology isn't *owned* by medical doctors, and that studying the nervous system means you can look at what parts of it are functioning properly… and the parts that *aren't!* The field of neuro*science* has bloomed since the late 90s, and doctors are now helping patients with conditions once thought untreatable!

He studied under Dr. Carrick- the neurologist who single-handedly changed concussion management when he resolved Pittsburgh Penguins hockey all-star Sid "The Kid" Crosby's lingering symptoms in a *month,* when no other team of "specialists" could, despite treating him for 9 *months*!

"The obvious example" Dr. Russ said, "is looking at stroke patients, because you can see exactly where an area is *damaged* in the brain… and therefore what weaknesses result from it. These can be studied. Well, now that we know about *neuroplasticity* and the brain's ability to wire and *re*-wire, we can also study *physiological* weaknesses or areas that *under*-perform (or *over*-fire in the cases of seizures)."

My jaw almost hit the floor right then and there! Was he suggesting that areas that aren't working right (but haven't been outright *damaged* - like from a stroke) can be re-wired to function more effectively, more normally?? Or even that stroke-damaged brains can re-wire the *healthy* areas to *compensate* for damage???

In fact, that's exactly what he meant. We started dating and having long, in-depth conversations about the nervous system. It was my passion, like working with children, but for my own selfish reasons! I wanted to be *normal!* I never knew what it felt like to be "normal."

I slowly began revealing my health secrets to him. Never trying to scare him off, always trying to see what he knew, and based on his experiences, what he believed was *possible!*

He had worked with many ADHD kids throughout his career, with some of the early pieces of neuroscience that could do the most good. He was big on nutrition, saying that "You are what you eat, but that applies to nutrients and junk food, not fat. Carbs make you fat. Sugar makes you fat. Not FAT."

The big moment came when he asked me innocently enough if I wanted to use what he knew to make some changes in myself? Did I want to use the newest neuroscience to modify my brain? Would I be willing to change my diet to support the growth of nerve cells and reduce inflammation?

It was almost like being asked to prom! I was completely nervous but excited at the same time. I wanted to get started right away! So he had me follow the lines on a piece of notebook paper with my eyes, and I felt my heart start to race uncontrollably!

He said that wasn't normal. I was having a fight or flight response to a simple brain challenge! (To this day, I still get a little pit in my stomach when he asks me to be the patient, to show parents what a healthy brain can do when following the stripes with the eyes. *And who'd have thought I would one day say I have a healthy brain???*)

He said that my brain was unstable. The right side of my brain was especially weak and *should* be able to follow a train going by or count moving stripes or walk past a picket fence without feeling jumpy while watching the posts).

So he began working with me. And I began working to improve my OWN brain. It was a lot of work, but not considering how much I had already been through.

And the differences started happening almost immediately!

I stopped passing out. My IBS (Irritable Bowel Syndrome) vanished. My memory returned (not of things that happened before my major seizure at age 20, but for everything new I was learning!) My eczema cleared up. I felt my coordination improve. The *radiculopathy* (nerve pains) in my shoulders and arms disappeared!

A month later, I felt like a new person. Transformed. Like being freed from my own body's prison!

THIS, after only a couple months before having been told I had a rare, incurable heart condition and that I should probably get a pacemaker. And just 4 years after having been told I was a good candidate for a *brain implant*!

Three months later, my neurologist took me off all my medications and released me from care! I was free.

The next month we began integrating some of these same therapies to my daughters to help with their grades and social skills. Except when there was head injury involved, my daughter hasn't had another seizure episode! I couldn't have been happier than to have one girl actually make it to the spelling bee and the other to be so happy and popular!

A few *more* months later, after endless training, and hundreds of hours of conversations with Dr. Russ, we started the MIND Institute for Neurological Development. Using what I learned with Dr. Russ, and applying it to the experience I gained working with all the learning disabled, behaviorally and developmentally challenged kids throughout the years, I realized that by missing out on life, by always being sick, that I wanted to change young lives for the better... so that they wouldn't have to go through what I did. A lifetime of pain and suffering.

Now that I understood the basis of neurological weakness, he helped me set a course to provide children (and adults) with a life of better moods, health, and brain function using the best tools and technology that exists on the planet.

I'm so happy with the positive changes we've made in clients' lives, I am finally optimistic about my future and the future of the lives we are able to reach!

PART 7 – DR. RUSS' STORY

Epilogue: by Dr. Russ

I had met Heather in fall of 2011, the week before I found out I had passed my Functional Neurology Fellowship. Two months before, I had flown down to Orlando, Florida where I met up with Dr. Jawad who I'd been studying with from Chicago. We sat and wrote our Boards for 5 straight hours in a room full of doctors, followed by giving a 30 minute presentation (recorded on video for other doctors to grade). Then we sat on our hands for 2 months, waiting for the results.

The week before I received my confirmation e-mail, I was (re)introduced to a Heather Bennett through a mutual friend. Now considering I didn't know a Heather Bennett in high school, it didn't surprise me to learn that her maiden name was Williams. I said maybe we should go out sometime and I would find her on facebook. (Dating sure has changed since we were in high school!)

When I met Heather for the first time since high school, I was shocked by her sincerity. "Most people just aren't this up-front about their feelings when they first meet" I thought.

She had her girls on a Sunday night, but we were able to meet up at Steak N' Shake. (Ever since my father's stroke back in 2009, I had made a commitment to take better care of myself, but for her, I thought I would let it slide. We ate burgers.)

We talked for what seemed like hours. We felt like old souls. I had asked during our very first texts to "give me the Cliff's Notes version of your life since high school."

What came back was a long list of uniquely original career choices, passions, and ideals. I definitely was impressed with her life. What came later was actually a shock. She said "I hope you don't think I'm trying to replace my neurologist with you."

I began to panic. The last person I dated who "had a neurologist" was bipolar and liked to throw things at my head! So I gently inquired "Why do *you* have a neurologist?"

She said softly "I was diagnosed with POTS and seizures years back." (Whew! I thought to myself. That I can deal with!)

It was only months and even *years* later that the story became more complete. The stories of doctors not believing her. The skin falling off and the hair falling out. I'll confess, I hadn't heard the term SJS (Stevens-Johnson Syndrome) but a couple of times prior to hearing Heather's story. I mean c'mon, it's a *one in a million* occurrence!

The injections below her skull. The radiculopathy. The passing-out spells. The IBS. The seizures. The heart condition she nearly had a pace-maker implanted for (just weeks before we met!)

I don't need to re-tell the story you just read, but I will tell you from my perspective, it was dumbfounding to hear what she had been through. Almost as equally incredible was that by taking a totally different perspective of her life and health, we were able to turn it all around in just a few short weeks.

We did some very basic, functional brain tests to see how her eye movements and coordination were. We looked at her over-all diet and beliefs on nutrition and turned them upside down.

We applied some very safe and simple techniques to help her brain to re-wire.

We took her off of the most processed, most dangerous foods in her diet. Goodbye to the gluten, beef jerky, and Mountain Dew! Hello Health!

And we changed her life. (I use the term "we" because my father, Dr. David Schroder, applied a few chiropractic alignments to her spine as needed. Plus, another functional neurologist, Dr. Gary

Smith, was there to back me up on some of the observations and clinical tests we made early on, during her initial work-up).

Most days I feel like we were fated to meet "again" when we did. (There is actually a picture of us IN Spanish class together!) If we'd known each other at Philo High School, though (before her BIG seizure, before she started her "new life" as a calmer person- with big chunks of memory loss), we may not have been right for each other (then). But today, with the conversations we've shared, our beliefs about over-prescription, our mutual goals for the future, the way we both enjoy helping people, I just feel blessed to have found her at this time in our lives.

She helped me to see what is possible- our role in the future of health care. My goal of a natural, non-drug system of re-wiring bad brains and healing inflammation damage is coming to life. She helped me see what we can really do for an individual and for a family.

I hope that you enjoy our story. Every bit of it is true. And we feel it is very powerful. It changed her life, and the lives of her family. And now, we are using it to help so many others!

2. NEUROLOGY 101

"We all agree that your theory is crazy, but is it crazy *enough*?" – Neils Bohr (Nobel Laureate – physics)

Neurology, as well as the field of Neuro*science*, is the study of the nervous system. The system of nerves that make up the human brain, spinal cord and peripheral nerves is vast, as there are more nerves in the brain than stars in the known galaxy. There are more connections in each and every human brain than there are grains of sand in the Mohave Desert.

In the next chapter we will draw out how the system of nerves are mapped out in your brain, connecting your body and the receptors feeding information from your body (back) to the brain. This is a tough chapter to approach considering it is so heavy in the language of neurology. It really is like learning a foreign language. It's time-consuming. And it will even be taxing on some injured brains that get tired reading a newspaper (written in language suited for a *sixth* grader).

This will be the heaviest chapter to read through and is really only meant to give some brief introductory concepts and language. The next chapter is for tracing along at home with a pen and paper. For now, we just ask that you bear with us as we take big leaps out of the gate to proceed quickly into the journey ahead.

To many neuroscientists the brain is thought of simply as a processing system or computer. This analogy is certainly preferable to no comparison at all, but as a metaphor it misses the fundamental and undeniable fact that the brain, spinal cord, and human nerves not only have the ability to change or rewire, but MUST wire and rewire as a God-given *right* in order to function at their ideal state.

The single immutable fact is that every one of us breathing oxygen right now on planet Earth is changing our brain on a daily basis with the actions we take, thoughts we think, and influences around us. In universities across the world, there are scientists testing theories, sharing data, and publishing research that looks at HOW our brains grow and develop- as well as what goes wrong to our precious three pound living computers that we all carry around in our skulls. (Kandel 2013)

Just how are we learning so much about the *human* brain since George H.W. Bush declared the 90s to be "THE Decade of the Brain" (back in 1989!)? Well, besides the anatomists who are slicing open cadavers and analyzing *which* pathways lead *where*, we also have neurologists who look at stroke patients and head-injury patients to find what *deficits* they have, based on *what area* was damaged. However, those have both been done for over 200 years! Here's a sample of what scientists are doing for the research of today and tomorrow!

Neuroscientists are:

- Putting patients into MRI machines and looking at the shapes and sizes of their brains

- Putting patients in MRI machines and injecting them with radioactively tagged glucose (sugar) molecules to see what parts of the brain light-up while performing certain actions

- Doing the same above while *thinking specific thoughts*

- Same as above while asked to *feel specific feelings*

- Hooking patients up to EEGs and measuring brainwaves in relaxed states, stressed states, while sleeping, while eating, and while drinking

- [Some neuroscientists work *specifically* for the food companies to test additives in food to find the *"sweet spot"* of flavor that lights up our brains the most (Moss 2013)]

- Performing spinal taps, drawing blood, or analyzing urine to look at neurotransmitters ("brain chemicals") and their metabolites (what they look like biochemically after they are broken down and filtered)

- Drawing blood to look at Vitamin D levels, Omega 3 levels, and inflammatory markers

- Zapping (with pulsed radio waves) different areas of the brain to temporarily turn them down (partially paralyze them) and measure for lost abilities

- Electrically stimulate different areas (like stimulating nerves with a TENS machine at the physical therapist's or chiropractor's office) to see what abilities are gained or lost

- Using computerized cameras for tracking eye movements of ADHD, Asperger's and Autistic children to see how they are *different* from the more typically developing children

- And *much, much more!*

All of this has lead to some pretty amazing discoveries. But at this point, we just want to stop and have you follow a few simple instructions. By doing this we know you will be lighting up certain areas of your brain.

First, get ready to close your eyes. Just blink and hold it for 3 seconds before you open them and continue reading.

Good. You just fired the 7th cranial nerve called the Facial nerve which sits in a part of the brainstem called the Pons. The connection it received from the brain sits in an area called Brodmann's area 4, the somatic motor strip (named after Korbinian Brodmann, a German neuroscientist who mapped out the different parts of the human cortex based on the cellular structures of the 6 layers of grey matter).

Still awake? That's because a part of the brainstem called the Mesencephalon (or simply mid-brain) is firing at a rate that's strong enough to keep your cortex activated to the point of consciousness. The brain in this state is firing Alpha or Beta waves when recorded on an EEG (Electro-encephalogram).

In the opposite situation, during sleep, the mid-brain fires *less* input to the thalamus first and then cortex as the brain gives off delta (slow) waves.

Lick your lips and shrug your shoulders. You just fired cranial nerve 11 and 12, the Spinal Accessory and Hypoglossal nerves that come out at the Medulla. (If we want to get technical, and just to show you how deep the rabbit hole goes the more you learn, the Spinal accessory nerve actually has its nuclei in the spinal cord down to about the 5th cervical vertebra, but it *exits* the central nervous system at the level of the Medulla and from within the skull... but you didn't need to know all that!)

Now, look quickly to the right side of the book. You just fired your left Frontal Eye Field (Brodmann's area 8 in the frontal lobe-sitting just inside your left temple). Quickly looking the opposite direction, left, fires the right frontal lobe.

You see the right side of the brain is concerned with information from the left side of the body and the left field of space. To see the right side of the brain "light up" on an fMRI (functional MRI- when the glucose is tagged), it's simply a matter of touching, moving, showing an image or making sound on the left side of the body. The type and strength of the input, determines how MUCH glucose the right hemisphere's cells drink up when they are firing.

Now, practice the piano with your right hand. Or tap your fingers rapidly and individually as if you were typing.

You just lit up a big chunk of the *left* brain/cortex and *right* cerebellum (a smaller more neuron-dense part of the brain involved with eye movements, accuracy and coordination of movements/ balance).

Here's where it gets interesting... Now, *IMAGINE* you are doing the right handed piano/typing exercise above. Do NOT move your fingers, but simply imagine it.

You just lit up the same neurons (nerve cells) in both parts of the brain listed above... just not as much!

In fact, if you even WATCH someone else type with their hand, those two same parts of your brain light up, but its mostly a specific type of cell called mirror-neurons!

How amazing is that?

Further research shows two other interesting points about how the brain works (and what happens when things go haywire).

1. If you were to practice playing the piano/typing in a controlled repetitive manner (a.k.a. if you "practiced"), not only would you become more proficient at it – you could "learn how to play the piano" or "learn to type" better and faster, but also *the nerve cells in those two specific areas of the brain would become denser* as the connections between them *grew and multiplied!*

2. The mirror-neurons mentioned above are drastically lacking in individuals on the Autism spectrum. These neurons are a form of feedback with the world. We can feel the tense-ness

OR elation in a room simply by observing the expressions or movements of the people in the room around us. Therefore those without the gift of mirror-neurons have been described as Mind-Blind. They have difficulty reading emotions of others. Hence they have trouble connecting and forming emotional bonds.

Now, if we combine the two points, we could logically conclude that by showing autistic patients our emotions more frequently or intensely (exaggerating our facial expressions), then the mirror-neurons could start to fire and grow connections so that they may come OUT of the mind-blindness.

This is an approach being used by parents and even tested by researchers across the globe. In fact, in the condition commonly referred to as dyslexia, reading programs are slowing down the speed at which words are processed. [We are said to be using BOTH of these approaches when we speak babytalk or "Motherese," with a very emotive and high pitch speech that includes drawing out the enunciation of words. This is a universal trait amongst mothers (and fathers, of course) in every culture]. (PBS 2002)

Many would say it's just a part of normal social (and emotional, AND educational development). The learning of language, and voice pitch, and bonding. So special, yet possibly overlooked by our internet, cell-phone, and hi-speed cable world.

Many things can happen to the system for it to go wrong, but let's pick a single example to represent what CAN and does happen hundreds of times a day (in a tribute to an old lecture also called "A Slip on the Ice.")

A SLIP ON THE ICE

A slip on the ice is a *small* thing. It happens hundreds of times a day.

A slip on the ice causes a man to fall and hit his head on the sidewalk. And that is a terrible thing... because-

That hit on the head causes the brain to shake inside of the skull as it bounces around in a watery cushion, but still within hard bone.

That bouncing around causes bruising and inflammation within the brain.

That inflammation within the brain activates a chemical cascade that continues and can even *grow* with a diet similar to the Standard American Diet (SAD).

That chemical cascade can even worsen if the head is hit again or the inflammatory SAD diet is continued for years.

That SAD diet is also laden heavily with sugars which are especially dangerous to nerve cells.

Now multiply that hit on the head, and/or inflamed SAD diet, or sugary nerve-damaging molecules times a thousand, and you affect the mental health and well-being of a town.

Multiply that hit on the head, and/or inflamed SAD diet, or sugary nerve-damaging molecules times a million, and you affect the mental health and well-being of a state.

Multiply that hit on the head, and/or inflamed SAD diet, or sugary nerve-damaging molecules times a 100 million, and you affect the mental health and well-being of a country.

Multiply that hit on the head, and/or inflamed SAD diet, or sugary nerve-damaging molecules times a billion, and you affect the mental health and well-being of the world.

And THAT, my friend, is a *very* big thing.

ADD/ADHD - A PARENT'S STORY

Last year, the doctor treated my son for hyperactivity with medications. He was disruptive in class and had trouble focusing. Over the summer I took him off the medication because I didn't want him on it year round because of the side-effects of those kind of drugs. Over the summer, I was getting ready for school, when they would probably tell me he needed to be put back on the medication so that he could focus in class and not interfere. But I met Dr. Russ Schroder and heard about his natural treatments for hyperactive kids and had him evaluated. We began treatment for my son. School started a couple weeks later and sure enough they suggested I go back to the meds, but I held out just a few more weeks. And I'm glad I did because when it came time for report cards and parent teacher conferences, they were nothing but excited about the progress that Jordan had made. His grades went up, and he was better behaved in class WITHOUT any meds.

3. THE NERVOUS SYSTEM

"Stated simply, it's a system of nerves."

Now that you made it through the big words in the last chapter, let's have some fun drawing!

We'll start with the side view of a brain. Draw a catcher's mitt on its side and then we will start filling in the other lines. Look at Figure 1.1. See how the T looks like the thumb of the mitt? The O is the heel. The P is the palm and the F makes up where the fingers would go! And the Cs line separates the palm from the fingers.

The F actually stands for the Frontal lobe of the brain. Keep in mind that as a side view, we are looking at one HALF of the brain, so it could be drawn in the opposite direction, too, as there are two hemispheres.

The Frontal lobe is involved with thinking, logic, reasoning, attention and sorting information/categorizing.

It has different parts to it as we alluded to earlier. The motor strip (M) is the part of the brain where, if we zapped it with an electrical probe, it would cause the related body part to move suddenly. The map on the brain represents the muscles under its control in the body. These areas can grow and shrink dramatically. They can even disappear or rewire to an entirely different body part in the instances of amputations! (Doidge 2007)

Its counterpart rests just behind here. On the other side of the Central Sulcus (valley) of Rolando (Cs) sits the Somatosensory strip (S) in the Parietal lobe (P). Zap here and you FEEL a place on your body where the sensory *map* represents.

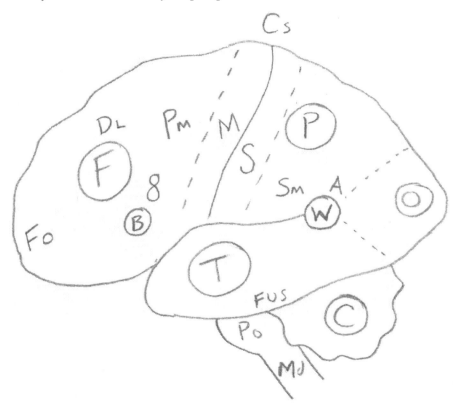

FIGURE 3.1   Left half of the brain/Left hemisphere
8= Brodmann's Area 8, A= Angular Gyrus, B= Broca's Area,
C= Cerebellum, Cs= Central Sulcus of Rolando, DL= Dorso-lateral Pre-
frontal Cortex, F= Frontal Lobe, Fo= Frontal-orbital/Fronto-polar
Cortex, Fus= Fusiform Gyrus, M= Motor strip, Md= Medulla,
O= Occipital Lobe, P= Parietal Lobe, Pm= Pre-motor Cortex, Po= Pons,
S= Sensory strip, Sm= Supra-marginal Gyrus, T= Temporal Lobe,
W= Wernicke's Area

Just in front of the motor strip is the Pre-Motor cortex (Pm). It is involved with the planning and coordination of movement. It sees that the rough draft or blueprints are being read by the motor strip and cerebellum (The C on the bottom right).

Remember that the cerebellum (Latin for "little brain") is a part of the brain involved with eye movements, accuracy, balance and coordination of movements. It controls the SAME side of the body. It is only 1/5th the size of the cerebral cortex, but it has 10X the number of nerve cells. It has been found in the last ten years to be a great processor. It has even been found to assist with the coordination of *thought!*

Getting back to the frontal lobe, our number 8 represents Brodmann's area 8, the Frontal Eye Fields mentioned previously. Turn the 8 on its side, and we can almost imagine a pair of eyes looking through glasses at us. If we fire this area with an electrical probe, the eyes will look to the opposite side of the body. So zapping the left 8 in the diagram, the eyes would move to the right. A more practical way to fire the area would be to just look quickly to the right!

Broca's area is illustrated by the big B. It is involved with spoken language. Damage here results in an expressive aphasia: the inability or difficulty speaking. It is Brodmann's area 44.

(Wernicke's area (W), also called Brodmann's are 22, sits in the temporal lobe. It is the receptive portion in our language system. Damage here can result in an inability to communicate because of not properly understanding language.)

The Frontal-orbital/ Frontal-polar region (Fo) is involved with long-term planning and other "Executive functions." *THE* classic case of what happens with *damage* here is Phineas Gage. He has been studied for over 100 years in neurology texts. He was a railroad worker who had a spike go straight through his Frontal pole region but survived. His doctor studied him and his new self. He lost the responsible traits of his character and became a spendthrift, drunk and gambler. They say "Gage wasn't Gage anymore."

In Figure 3.2, we can look down at the brain. The Occipital lobes (O), sit in the very back portion receiving vision impulses from the receptors in the eyes (called rods and cones). From above, the brain can be drawn much like a football split in half, with the parietal lobes separating the frontal and occipital lobes.

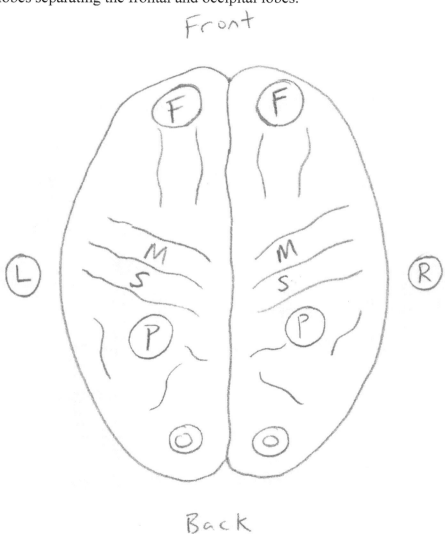

FIGURE 3.2 Top view of the brain/ The brain from above.
F= Frontal Lobes, L= Left, M= Motor strip, P= Parietal Lobes,
O= Occipital Lobes, R= Right, S= Sensory strip

(Back in Figure 3.1) The Dorso-lateral Pre-frontal cortex (DL) is involved with sorting, categorizing and organizing new information.

The left Angular gyrus (A) is involved with math, metaphors, and abstract thinking. The right is involved with our sense of space in relation to others.

The Supramarginal gyrus (SM) is important in the sequencing of movements. Damage here causes a multitude of *dyspraxias,* or inabilities to perform complex movements- like opening a pickle jar, combing our hair or brushing our teeth.

The Temporal Lobes (T) are specialized for higher functions like long-term memory, hearing, and emotions. The Fusiform gyrus sits on the bottom half. (Fus below) Damage to this area results in an inability to distinguish fine details or recognize faces (a condition called *prosopagnosia*).

Figure 3.3 is the inside of the right half of the brain. It always reminds me of a big puffy cloud on a stick. The Thalamus (Th) sits deep in the brain. There is one per hemisphere. Each thalamus is a junction box for the senses. Think of it as a great train station that takes in all the senses (except smell) before they are sent to the lobes of the brain. Stroke damage here has caused patients to be in pain on the entire opposite side of their body.

The Anterior Cingulate Gyrus (ACG) sits on the inner wall of the brain. It is a part of the frontal lobe. It is involved with our basic drives and motivation as well as empathy. Weakness here can cause a lack of motivation or a lack of empathy.

The Corpus Callosum (CC) is the "great bridge" between the left and right hemispheres. It is made up of 200 million nerve fibers connecting the paired areas of the human cortex together. (e.g. left and right frontal lobes) The corpus callosum is larger in women than men. An extremely rare condition called *agenesis of the corpus callosum* results in one big hemisphere. Kim Peek (the basis of Dustin Hoffman's *Rain Man* character) had this. He couldn't forget any information he read. But it also caused obvious social deficits.

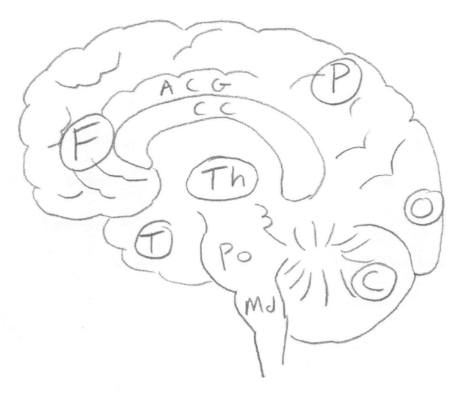

FIGURE 3.3   Inside view of the right brain/ Right hemisphere
ACG= Anterior Cingulate Gyrus, C= Cerebellum, CC= Corpus
Callosum, F= Frontal Lobe, Md= Medulla, O= Occipital Lobe,
P= Parietal Lobe, Po= Pons, T= Temporal Lobe, Th= Thalamus
The Mid-brain (unlabeled) sits between the Pons and the thalamus.

The Medulla (Md) sits at the very top of the spinal cord. It is the bottom third of the brainstem It's home to cranial nerves 9,10,11, and 12. It's involved with moving the tongue, digestion, swallowing, the regulation of digestion and heart rate, and shrugging the shoulders.

The Pons (Po) sits above the Medulla in the brainstem. It is home to cranial nerves 5,6,7, and 8. Therefore, it's major functions are moving the eyes laterally (outward) under the control of the cortex, feeling and moving the face, salivating, producing tears, balance, hearing, and taste.

An area called the Ponto-medullary reticular formation (PMRF) here in the lower 2/3rds of the brainstem help regulate pain, blood vessel tone, sweat glands, and muscle tone on the same side of the body. *NINETY* percent of the cortex of the human brain (the *neo-*cortex- because it's so new to develop) fires down to this region to help with blood flow to the gut, reduced pain reception and muscle tone for ease of posture.

The Mesencephalon (mid-brain) is a very small portion of the brainstem that sits just above the pons. It is involved with our waking states and processing intensity of light. It constricts the pupils of the eyes. Damage here could cause a large pupil (the reason they shine light in a patient's eyes at the ER to see if someone has a concussion) The 3rd and fourth cranial nerves reside here and move the eye muscles.

The Reticular Activating System in the mesencephalon is involved with keeping us awake and alert. Damage here is most evident in coma patients or patients in "persistent vegetative states" who may actually be firing brain-waves, but whose brains aren't stable enough to awaken. There has been tremendous interest in this field in the past few years alone. Doctors are utilizing brain-based techniques to gently start pushing the weak areas to fire at a slightly higher rate, and even to wake from comas!

For Figure 3.4, draw some bottom teeth with the roots (dots) inside connecting to a dot in another tooth and one deep below. The dots actually represent neurons. The ones in the teeth are part of the *gray matter* of the cortex. The one deep below is in one of the deep structures of the brain. The short and long range wires (axons) connect local or distant regions of the brain. A long tract called the *arcuate fasciculus* actually connects Wernicke's to Broca's area.

Diffusion tensor imaging, a new type of MRI, is an exciting new technology that shows how the tracts can be weak, under-developed, or flat-out damaged from trauma.

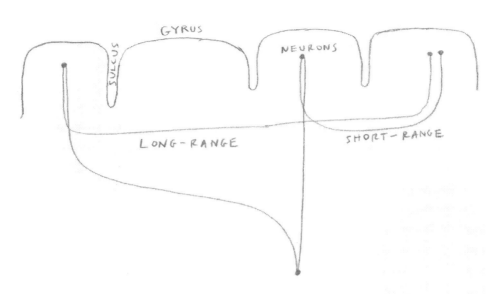

FIGURE 3.4   The brain's connections/ slice of the Cerebral Cortex. What's under the surface. Includes Short Range and Long Range connections (axons) between neurons, Gyrus is a ridge (Gyri plural), Sulcus is a groove (Sulci plural)

PROBLEMS

On the following pages, we list some of the most common problems that occur in the brain. Our genetics *do* contribute, but they represent only a *fraction* of the cases. More importantly, we now have a better understanding about how our genes are influenced by our *diet and lifestyles!* (Hyman 2003) Some problems are multi-factorial. Others we are still learning about have come a long way since the 70's when our parents were in school.

1. Inflammation- Time magazine had a cover article called The Fires Within as far back as 2004 that addressed the enormous challenges that an inflamed nation is up against health-wise.

   Since inflammation is linked to all chronic degenerative conditions, many children born to inflamed mothers are already epigenetically starting off with genes set to express an inflamed body.

2. High sugar/high carbohydrate diets- 1/3rd of African-Americans will be diabetic (type 2) by the age of 18. Type 2 diabetes *used* to be called "Adult-onset" but that becomes contradictory when so many children are obese/diabetic.
   Let's not ignore the ever present fact that a fasting blood sugar must be 127 to be labeled diabetes, but under 100 is normal.

   The forgotten part is that *100- 126 is not normal.* It means the body has developed insulin resistance. The receptors on the cells have become numb to insulin molecules. This is called pre-diabetes, and the world should take note because it is a global problem.

   (In Kuwait, they are calling it "The OTHER Gulf War Syndrome" because the American-ization of the middle eastern diet has now made 80% of Kuwait's population pre-diabetic or diabetic!

3. Auto-immune disorders- becoming much more common. In The Autoimmune Epidemic (Nakazawa 2008) we are told about the NIH and CDC's newest in-depth studies at how our immune systems are attacking our own bodies! The immune reaction is inflammatory, so this is a big overlap to #1 above.

4. Food sensitivities- these are rampant. It used to be the odd kid in school who couldn't be near peanuts or was lactose intolerant. Now waves of children are being tested by immunologists. Their blood can be drawn and markers for reaction to the proteins in food can be measured.

What's coming out is astounding! We are reacting, and over-reacting to the very foods that dominate our food supply. Children have gluten, dairy, corn, and soy sensitivities to name a few. A quick Google search of "GF DF SF" (gluten-free, dairy-free, soy-free) finds entire communities of people "going paleo" – or getting back to the nutrition of our hunter-gatherer ancestors who wouldn't dare try to sneak up on a wild cow to suckle its milk. And try tasting some wheat fresh off the stalk. Not very enjoyable, therefore not eaten except when near starvation!

5. Head injuries- when our heads hit something hard, or when we have them in a helmet, but the *helmet* hits something hard. When our brains bounce around inside a skull that has some pointy areas in it. And worst, when we send our little boys out as young as age four and tell them to go run into the other boys (as if their brains were even fully developed!).

These are the repetitive minor but cumulative bumps that tear the nerve cells in the brain microscopically, causing inflammation to prevent infection. It was said that Hall-of-Fame defensive back, Junior Seau never got knocked out throughout his entire 17 year NFL career. He said he never had a concussion in high school or college either!

But when they opened him up during his autopsy, after he shot himself in the chest, they found CTE, Chronic Traumatic Encephalopathy- a neurodegenerative disorder caused by humans banging their heads together repeatedly. (And in fighters who at least have the decency to use their fists to try to knock a man down.!

6. Nutritional deficiencies- More than 92% of Americans are deficient in *at least* one vitamin or mineral. (Hyman 2009) Our food supply has been grown on the same soil now for decades. It isn't as mineral or nutrient rich as it once was.

7. Even Worse... THE PRODUCTS WE PUT *INTO* OUR FOOD SUPPLY! – There is a frightening website that details all the ways in which the food manufacturers sneak MSG (or at least the reactive part, the "free glutamic acid" into our food and drinks. It's TruthInLabeling.Org. Go there. Soon.

Canned soups. Jerky. Snacking peanuts. Breads. Prepared meats. Flavorings. Additives. It's almost ubiquitous in the Standard American Diet.

The problem... MSG is an *excitotoxin!* (Blaylock 1996) It exists in small doses in the human body and is released and absorbed by nerve cells. But too much of a "good thing" is a very *very* bad thing. Prior to World War II, this wasn't found in the world's food supply. The U.S. soldiers wondered why the Japanese rations tasted so good. They had a secret ingredient. MSG.

It became so popular that the federal government approved it easily enough and is even considered "Natural" when a health conscious person eats it in an all-natural snack! Go to the website above and read the over *three dozen* different names they have used for MSG! ... Or simply go to a Doritos bag and you'll see a handful of them!

8. Functional Disconnections/Physiological Lesions- there are numerous terms used to describe weakened/ poor/ abnormal communication connections in the central nervous system. Some call them "physiological abnormalities" and others simply "functional changes." (Moller 2006)

In patients with a cast on an arm or leg, on MRI, the cortex will be thinner in areas that control or sense that body part. This happens in chronic pain states and limb amputations as well. So, some researchers even refer to this as "gray matter decrease" or "cortical thinning." (UCLA researchers found in 2009 that cortical thinning is widespread in ADHD!)

Since the brain is so highly malleable and re-wiring can and does occur, whether we like it or not, we must abide by the most natural developmental principles available.

In regards to relative importance of developmental milestones, all are significant in some way. Not learning to hold our head up soon enough means the wiring between the neck and the eyes (the VOR, Vestibulo-Ocular Reflex- "Welcome back neurology!") is poor in developing. Children in Eastern Bloc, Russian, and Chinese nurseries and institutions who aren't held or petted and "cooed at," in the way mothers and fathers were designed to do, have bonding issues. Some of them don't even grow the bonding center in the brain (The ACC- anterior cingulated cortex).

Functional Disconnections were discovered shortly after *permanent* disconnections were discovered (created) by neurologists at USC in the 50's. In an effort to prevent the spread of seizures in the brain, they sliced parts of the brain apart from the rest, separating the connections. (They got the idea from firefighters who prevent the spread of forest fires by preventatively burning a healthy strip of trees to create a barrier the fire can't pass). Roger Sperry won the Nobel Prize for his work on split-brain studies after they began noticing the subtle but significant differences in a patient's brain when it isn't wired properly… when it is disconnected!

The disconnections/weak firing/functional changes lead to timing issues, or "temporal binding", or even "temporal processing issues." These are brains that haven't developed properly in their wiring, most typically. It is studied heavily these days by EEG, fMRI, and SPECT scans in patients with ADHD, Autism, Reading problems and many other types of neurological disorders. (Melillo 2005)

AUTISM

Our son is 6 and was diagnosed a few years ago with High-functioning Autism. Before starting, our son would have a meltdown everyday over very small things. Things as small as dropping a pencil would cause him to spiral into a meltdown. He was also a very picky eater and never tried anything new. His imaginative play was very limited.

Our son would ask the same question over and over again, almost as if he did not remember he had already asked the question. He would have a really hard time going to sleep and staying asleep. We have been giving him melatonin at night to help him get to sleep and have for the last couple years.

After we started at the MIND Institute, within just a couple of weeks we were noticing small changes in him. His imaginative play had increased tremendously. He was asking to try more foods. We were noticing less meltdowns over little things.

After a couple months, we were no longer giving him the melatonin every night to help him get to sleep. He was now getting tired and falling asleep on his own more often. He has become more daring, like a little boy, and climbs on things, jumps off of things and does other things that other boys would typically do.

Our son has become more comfortable with others and does not seem to have the anxiety that he did have. His personality has changed to become more age appropriate. The training sessions have helped our son on so many levels. I get excited to see him doing new things, changing and maturing into a little boy.

It is so exciting to see him playing *with* other kids, not just alongside, and socializing not just with kids but whoever he is around.

ATTENTION ISSUES

My son has a lack of attention and focus issues with school. He has poor organization skills and therefore loses important papers to complete. He is getting poor grades. Currently, he is using the Neuro Integrator. He is about half way through the sessions... His organization has gotten much better, and he has not lost *any* school papers. He remembers when his tests are so I can help him study. He also seems to stay on task or topic easier instead of jumping around.

4. ADD/ADHD

"Labels are for cans, not people."

In 2013, we had the experience of working with numerous children labeled ADD or ADHD. (Author's note: ADHD will be the catch-all term used here to "label" those with the attention deficit disorder with OR without the hyperactivity component.)

It was a very busy year for us as we made a lot of important distinctions about how children are treated locally. It was frightening actually. The shear number of medications that are being forced on children by the pharmaceutical companies is staggering to say the least.

As we noted in the Introduction, two key points are noteworthy.

1. Childhood mental disorders are on the rise

2. Medications used to treat ADHD *cause* bipolar disorder and other problems (Whitaker 2010)

It was hard to find a child who was on "just" one medication for their ADHD. Most were on at least two. Several were on 3 or MORE!

And it was also shocking the TYPE of medications they were using to treat ADHD. A *dangerous, illegal*, and growing trend in the U.S. is for drug manufacturers to push doctors to write prescriptions for anti-psychotics for ADHD "*off*-label." (see Chapter 7)

Abilify and Risperdal are anti-psychotics which are approved to treat bipolar disorder, schizophrenia, other serious mental problems and irritability related to autism. However they are not FDA Approved for ADHD or other neuro-behavioral problems of childhood... meaning they are being written *off*-label. But some children were being prescribed them as a secondary medication besides drugs like Ritalin, Adderall, Straterra or Metadate (methylphenidate).

We wondered, was this in an effort to complement the effects of the legal ADHD drugs? ... or possibly to *reduce or counteract the side-effects of the ADHD drugs!*

A government study came out in November of 2013 saying that over 10% of kids have been given the ADHD label. That makes for a LOT of prescription sales! Billions of dollars worth in fact. It doesn't help that some of the "ADD support groups" are really fronts for the drug companies. It's no coincidence that their recommended treatments of choice just *happen* to be the very drugs the company makes! CHADD is one example. (Selling Sickness 2005)

All of this is at the expense of what research has to say about some of the *causes* of ADHD as well as what other *non-*pharmaceutical interventions have the ability to do!

Multiple studies have shown that ADHD is actually found with a thinned cortex of the brain (a functional disconnection or a *delay* in the maturing of the cortex) in the frontal lobes, primarily the right hemisphere. Research as far back as 1986 to today, from such sources as Yale and Harvard, has documented this rather conclusively. (American Journal of Psychiatry 1986/ Journal of Learning Disabilities 2000/ Journal of Pediatrics 2009)

Numerous studies have shown that ADHD (as well as mental health risks) is directly related to low levels of essential fats in the blood. We are not talking about Omega 6's, that's for sure! Our diet is loaded in inflammatory Omega 6's... From corn and soy to wheat and other grains!

Instead, we are talking about Omega 3 essential fats, primarily DHA and EPA, (Docosahexaenoic Acid and Eicosapentaenoic Acid) found almost exclusively in fish. Since our water supply isn't ideal, (and since the authors aren't big fans of the *flavor* of most fish), supplementation is common and may even be the ideal in the future. (It was just 3 years ago that Japan had an environmental mess with their nuclear plant dumping radiation into the Pacific ocean). Tuna has minimal omega 3s (and is packaged in cans lined with questionable man-made chemicals).

Breastfeeding dramatically reduces the risk of ADHD (and ear infections as well.) (Perlmutter 2006)

Reducing TV time can result in a significant reduction in ADHD symptoms. (Martin 2011) The flashing images that scroll across our children's eyes directly bypass the rest of the brain involved with sensation and exercise and go straight through a gateway station (the thalamus) to the visual cortex. This means their brain gets stimulated without having to move. Normally we "wire in" coordination and movement while we get visual stimulation. TV *bypasses* that. Even video-games only fire to the hands (true, there is *some* hand-eye coordination) but not the rest of the motor system. So we get brain stimulation without the outlet of movement (the inverse of running or playing). In essence, the toy train is "wound up" but not released to travel.

As you will see in chapter 9, with excitotoxins found almost everywhere in our food supply, the brain is being (over)fired just with the "food" we eat. And I say food with quotes because an ancestor of ours wouldn't even recognize most of what we eat now as being edible (until he took the first bite and got hooked by the flavor!)

This is actually how drug-dealers and tobacco manufacturers drum up business. Fire up the pleasure centers of the brain. Cause it to release dopamine. And watch the desire soar. And we all know *drugs* are addictive…How about our foods!?

The British journal *Lancet* found in 2004 that food colorings and benzoate preservatives caused a relative *increase* in hyperactivity symptoms that was *directly related to the amount consumed.*

They concluded that the additives are of concern, not just because of the rise in ADHD children, but because they represent a public health issue, having an overall "detrimental effect on children's behavior." This being the case, ''…if additives have an effect at all, it is via a *pharmacological* effect''!

This is exactly the point David Kessler makes in The End of Overeating. The former FDA head, who went after big tobacco in the 90's, points out in his book that food manufacturers use a number of different tricks and countless chemicals to trick the taste-buds, increase appetite and stimulate the release of dopamine.

There is a vast wealth of research regarding Neurofeedback for ADHD. Most research now is clearly pointing to ADHD as being a an issue with the cortical wiring of the brain- with most children who are diagnosed showing "neurological soft-signs." (Developmental Neuropsychology 2010) These are weaknesses in the brain that have been mentioned throughout this book.

Testing strongly shows weaknesses of the frontal lobes or right brain. (Neuropsychiatry 2000) This includes motor performance and eye movements besides EEG activity. (Journal of Neurophysiology 2003)

Several books reference dozens of studies dating back to the 80's including Getting Started With Neurofeedback, A Symphony in the Brain, and the Handbook of Neurofeedback.

In Newsweek, all the way back in June of 2000, researchers said;

"The technology is still in its infancy [back in 2000], but its emerging as a tool to treat everything from epilepsy and ADHD to migraines, anxiety, depression, head injuries, sleep disorders and even addiction. In the last few years, neurofeedback has made its way into the offices of hundreds of reputable doctors, psychologists and counselors."

Even Dr. Russell Barkley, a psychiatrist at the Medical University of South Carolina who was *highly* skeptical at first, was persuaded to look at the latest available research showing "significant reductions in impulsiveness and inattention."

All the way back in 2001, in his book Healing ADD, Daniel Amen gave neurofeedback protocols for the different types of ADD/ADHD, as well as warning against sugary processed foods. He is someone with experience. As the head of the Amen Clinics (and frequent contributor to PBS specials on brain health), he is the world's leading researcher in PET scans of the brain, having analyzed tens of thousands over the past 20 years!

The MIND Method utilizes neurofeedback, neurological testing, the Interactive Metronome and nutrition as cornerstones for children with ADHD (and yes, ADD for clarification).

Our non-drug, natural approach to finding weak areas of the brain has helped countless children and families to achieve higher grades, better social skills, and improved coordination. Tracking neurological improvement has never been easier with the latest technologies.

We, too, are tired of the dangerous trends in medicine, with drug companies controlling *half* of the budget of the FDA. (Angell 2005) The British medical journal the *Lancet* said back in 2002, the FDA is "highly vulnerable to … conflicts of interests." Or basically that the drug companies are paying off regulators, researchers, and even the very doctors that prescribe their drugs, through paid trips, gifts and free dinners.

ADHD- BEYOND THE MEDS

My son is 10 years old and I've noticed issues with him since he was about two year old. I've been dealing with him behavior-wise since about that age, and as he became older, pre-school age. Behavior was getting worse (despite numerous doctors and medications.) Learning disabilities were taking place at this time. At an IEP meeting, a teacher suggest that I have him neurologically tested. Just that week I read a post about the MIND Institute on Facebook and thought "This might be an answer!" They tested him, showed what they were looking for specifically, and we began his training.

Now, in school, my son's behavior is better. He has avoided several fights, whereas before he used to chime in on them. Now, he's standing on the sidelines, which is a big plus. You have to earn the rights to go on field trips which he has done now. I've pointed this out to him and praised him for it. All because we're going to the MIND Institute.

His teacher lets him know "You're doing great. We're seeing some good changes." And GRADES HAVE COME UP! I'm amazed that his grades have come up. He's got A's and B's! His last report card, last quarter, which was before we started coming to the MIND Institute was C's and D's.

I was amazed that last Friday, he brought books home. He's wanting to read more! I was just so happy that he brought like 5 books home to read. And so far today, he has already read 2 of them.

All of this is with less medication! He has been on medication since he was 4 (and he's 10 now). He's been on different ones, different doses. Nothing seems to have helped... until now. I guess you could say it's been a blessing from God.

BEHAVIOR ISSUES

My son had just turned 14 when we started [at the MIND Institute]. His history is that at 4 he started having seizures, he would not talk to other people, family only. Diagnosed with severe anxiety, mild autism, borderline Developmental Disabilities. He did grow out of seizures at 12 years old. He started therapy and diet a month before school started. After two weeks of school, I heard comments like "Dale's a new man." Teachers said he was behaving better. He only needs one re-direction to behave. before it was re-direct, re-direct, re-direct until he was out in the hall. Changing his diet and therapy have improved his mood and mood swings tremendously. He was not able to deal with disappointment or change very well, had meltdowns and was violent. We've had NO violent behavior and since second or third month- NO meltdowns. We have taken him off one medication, with no problems, ready to remove the last med. He will look people in the eye and speak back to them now. He still has a hard time with impulse control, but it is a LOT better. I think he will keep improving!

FROM OUR STAFF

Since starting at the MIND Institute last year, I have been amazed to see the tremendous amount of progress that occurs in the kids. I work with the children who are mildly to severely autistic as well as those with ADHD and behavioral problems. There has been immense change in their behavior! They have all been performing better in school, as well as when they come in for their training. Their communication is enhanced. They are starting to develop the ability to converse with others and have started bonding with me and their parents! I feel blessed to work with such clients and families that are ready for positive changes without all the stress!

- Hailey George

5. DYSLEXIA

"Readin, Rightin, and Rithmetic"

No longer is the focus of education on just helping children get good grades. More and more colleges are relying on tests like the SATs and ACTs to hand-pick which children they want to take from young-adult to adult in their prestigious and expensive establishments.

Plus, it is becoming more difficult for teachers to have lasting and personal interactions with children due to growing class sizes, decreased pay, and an ever-present quota in the new national conundrum of standardized tests.

Now teachers are finding themselves teaching to the tests while entire school districts in parts of the U.S. are being caught *cheating*. Entire boxes of scan-tron tests sheets are found to have "too high of a rate of erasure corrections"- meaning that it is normal to have students erase answers and change them. However, there is a reasonable number of answers that will be changed for the right answer (just like answers will be changed for the *wrong* answer, too.

Some school districts just have a disproportionate number of students who have the wrong answer initially but then correct themselves. Or another way of saying it- the teachers and administrators are the cheaters!

We all want our children to do well. We want them to get good grades, stay in school so they can get a good education and not spend their lives working hard for little pay. It's what our grandparents and parents did for us (hopefully!).

Problems arrive when executive areas of the brain don't process information properly, though. Especially on the left side of the brain.

Over 150 years ago in Europe there were two neurologists who found two separate and distinct areas of the brain on the left side that are BOTH involved with speech and language.

Drs. Paul Broca and Karl Wernicke will be remembered to this day because they both had patients with strokes that survived long enough that they could examine them thoroughly before their ultimate autopsy at death. (You will remember them from chapter 3 for their named regions on the cortex of the brain.) Each one found that the individual they examined for language/speech challenges had a big gaping blood clot in the left hemisphere. Of course, this was in the 1800's, long before MRIs showed us *functional* weaknesses. Back then they were lucky to have such obvious examples of pathology so the world could start to learn that different regions serve different functions!

A hundred and thirty years later, science began to look inside the brains of patients with strokes and tumors *without* cutting them open, and similar patterns began to emerge.

In Sally Shaywitz's book, Overcoming Dyslexia, we learn of her research at Yale where they took numerous children and adults with Developmental Reading Disorders (a.k.a. Dyslexia), and put them in PET scanners and fMRI scanners with tagged glucose. What they found over and over was weakness on the left side of the brain in areas between Wernicke's area (the parietal/occipital/temporal junction) and Broca's area of the frontal lobe.

She also found that most children with dyslexia have normal and even-above average intelligence. They don't have vision problems that cause the reading disorder. But many describe the "shapes and symbols" made up of letters and words to be "reversed" or upside down. They find b and d are easily transposed. As are p and q. Since they are essentially the same shape, just pointing in different directions, a mis-firing cortex can't interpret them correctly.

Even tractography studies (that look at the long tracts or long-*range* nerve connections) show weaknesses on the left side of the brain. (*Brain* 2012)

In The Woman Who Changed Her Brain, Barbara Arrowsmith-Young discusses the learning disabilities she suffered with until her adult life regarding shapes and words. Through painstaking months of slow, deliberate work, she studied the works of Alexandr Luria, a Russian neuroscientist who had the privilege of studying hundreds of Russian soldiers with head injuries (even bullet wounds!) in specific *regions of the brain.*

She found the case of a soldier who had her symptoms and actually had a bullet wound in a very specific area of the brain, the left parietal cortex. Through neurological training, she performed exercises that forced her to develop that weakened area in her brain. She went on to form numerous schools in Canada that use brain exercises to help children with reading and learning disorders. (Eaton 2011) (American researchers have been utilizing Neurofeedback more often for learning deficiencies since the 80's).

It's even been found that stuttering also correlates with weakness of the tracts or cortex of the left brain (Neurology 2003) These children also have the hope of benefit from re-wiring the brain.

Our approach has always been to build up the weak areas *after* a thorough exam. We have also seen weaknesses on the left side of the brain that correlate with some of the functional weakness on the right side of the body. (*BMC Neuroscience* 2009)

Therapies include nutritional strategies to support normal nerve connections, neurological activities like eye-exercises and the Interactive Metronome, plus another go-to is Neuro-Integration (neurofeedback with visual entrainment).

DYSLEXIA

When I first heard about Dr. Russ's program for Dyslexia I had been suffering for the past several months with reading and concentration difficulties. It seemed ridiculous to me that as a grown man and an avid reader, I would just START to suffer with problems like this. But I couldn't finish a book. I was distracted. Plus the words were starting to become jumbled and run together. I was really becoming depressed about it.

But everything that I heard Dr. Russ say made sense from a brain perspective. When I saw him, he took a thorough history and did a very specific exam relating to my focus problem. He noticed some very obvious problems on the tests. Heck, even I could see and feel some of the findings. (With my eyes closed, my balance was WAY off.)

He accepted me for treatment, I started care and looking back, I realize that just a few short weeks later, I had read *Brave New World* and several other books in just a couple months time WITHOUT DIFFICULTY! I highly recommend Dr. Russ Schroder and his program!

6. AUTISM

"She herself faces, almost every day, extreme variations,
from overresponse to underresponse, in her own sensory
system"
- Oliver Sacks, about Temple Grandin,
from *An Anthropologist on Mars*

In the 1940s, two physicians, Leo Kanner and Hans Asperger, in two different parts of the world were both discovering a condition that would later be labeled as Autism (spectrum disorders).

Autism is a neuro-developmental disorder that is diagnosed after 3 basic criteria are observed.

1. Impairment of social interactions (social withdrawal)

2. Impairment of communication with others (verbal and non-verbal)

3. Impairment of play and imaginative activities (frequently seen as repetitive behaviors)

(Dr. Asperger had a thorough understanding of the varied *spectrum* of characteristics that are seen. Therefore what will now be called "High functioning autism," in the new "DSM-5," was previously labeled "Asperger's syndrome.")

There are a wide range of symptoms and behaviors that are common along with this triad of impairments. These include:

- Spasms, tics, twitches
- Rocking back and forth
- Hand-wringing, hand-flapping
- Poor eye-contact
- Dietary difficulties (limited range of food choices)
- Exaggerated sensory responses *or* reduced responses (reduced or increased pain perception/hearing/ taste)
- Paradoxical sensory responses (some heightened with others reduced)

What is most frightening about the diagnosis is that there are more and more children being seen who have theses traits each year. In every state, in every region of the world, there are more children who have the characteristics and traits that fit the diagnosis (label) "autistic."

In 1970, few doctors or patients had heard of autism. Only about 1 in 10,000 children were diagnosed. By 1995, 1 in 500 were found to be on the spectrum. By 2002 it was 1 in 150. In 2006, 1 in 110. In 2011, about 1 in 88. And in 2013, large population studies were showing 1 in 50!

FRIGHTENING STATISTICS

Nearly half of all autistic children will run away or go missing before they even turn 17. (ABC News 5/2/13/ American Academy of Pediatrics) This is often referred to as "eloping" by clinicians.

To family members and neighbors, it is more commonly referred to as "a nightmare" as many of these children never make it home. It is a relief to everyone involved when they DO come home safe and sound, but *when they don't, the statistics say* that 9 times out of 10, they will *drown.*

All the more important that the medical establishment needs to shrug off the "label and drug" mindset that limits the effective management and often reversal of the condition through *brain-based* therapies and exercises. (Melillo 2012)

Going further upstream in the events of causation, many researchers even argue that a proper focus on *prevention* is critical. For instance many women have difficulty even having a baby when they have a low thyroid. Many have secondary issues like PCOS (Polycystic ovarian syndrome) as well. (Kharrazian 2010)

But it is indeed important to address the state of the mother's health, as a hypothyroid mother is *FOUR TIMES* more likely to "produce autistic children" than healthier women! (ScienceDaily 8/13/13)

Neurofeedback, other brain-based therapies, and nutritional approaches have shown great benefit for many children (and adults) on the spectrum. (Evans 2007) Behavioral-based treatments like the Son-Rise program were some of the first to show that autism *is* actually reversible in many cases. These are time-intensive, but at least they showed that having hope is not irrational, but actually beneficial. Hope means parents will *do what it takes* to get results.

The Brain-Balance centers are another example of brain-based treatments. Having trained with the founder, Dr. Robert Melillo, we've modeled much of our kids' functional training on his procedures, but we place an even bigger emphasis on Neurofeedback, nutrition, and inflammation management (everything listed in the Q and A section of Chapter 10). Dr. Melillo has been a strong advocate for autism treatment in general, and has authored 4 books on Autism and other neuro-behavioral disorders.

AUTISM SPECTRUM

Our son was diagnosed with mild autism in the summer time last year. We first noticed some things with him before he turned 4 years old that were concerning. We were referred up to Children's where our assumptions were confirmed with him going up there and being diagnosed at the CDC [Centers for Disease Control], going through all their tests, which is a pretty long process (about 4 hours for a couple different sessions where they sit down with him).

He wasn't talking very much He wasn't doing some of the things that he SHOULD do for his age, being four years old.

Really, he's been coming- to boost his deficiencies, you could say, with his mind. We didn't want to do any kind of medication.

We just wanted him to be more like every other kid. And we have been getting there, and his therapies here have been helping out A LOT. He really likes to come down [to the MIND Institute]. He looks forward to coming down and doing his different exercises. His coordination is a lot better. His speech has improved.

I think it's definitely because he comes here a good bit (in combination with his other therapies and tutors at school). He's really made a lot of progress in the past 5 months.

With his speech he was only saying a few words, very limited speech. No where near what it should have been for his age. He wasn't even really asking basic questions. He was having a hard time telling you what he wanted sometimes. We'd ask "Do you want this?" and he would just cry out, he wouldn't tell you what he wanted. Now you'll ask him what he wants and he'll tell you or he'll go get it himself sometimes or he'll point to it and say "I want that up there." He's gotten a lot better about that. A lot of stuff he just gets himself anymore. A lot of times with breakfast, he'll put his bowl and spoon in the sink without being told.

He's asking more questions, like "who what why when and how?" Before he wasn't asking anything like that, he was only using a couple words in conjunction. It wasn't any full sentences.

We're very pleased with what he's been doing combined with his other therapies, and without medication. They're looking now to even move him into more of a standard classroom, where they do more normal schoolwork. They think now he can really benefit from that because he's been making SUCH good progress the last few months.

He's really come a long way from not talking a whole lot, not being able to do a whole lot of tasks without a lot of help. He's definitely moved in leaps and bounds here over the last few months. His time here has definitely been a large impact on that.

7. ANXIETY/ DEPRESSION/ BIPOLAR

"Before I built a wall I'd ask to know
What I was walling in or walling out."
- Robert Frost, *Mending Wall*

In 2012, after a 7 year investigation, GlaxoSmithKline (GSK) was fined $3,000,000,000 (3 BILLION dollars) by the federal government for the company's illegal promotion of its medications- the largest fine ever levied on a drug company. (AP Newswire 7/1/12)

Were they selling their drugs' secrets to the Nazis or Osama Bin Laden?

No, instead, GSK illegally promoted the drug Paxil for treating depression in children from April 1998 to August 2003, even though it was NEVER approved by the FDA for anyone under the age of 18. They also promoted the drug Wellbutrin from January 1999 to December 2003 for weight loss, the treatment of sexual dysfunction, substance addictions and ADHD, even though it was only approved for treatment of major depressive disorder.

In fact, it is 100% ILLEGAL to promote uses for a drug that have not been approved by the FDA- a practice known as *OFF-Label Marketing*.

At the press conference after the verdict Acting Assistant Attorney General Stuart F. Delery, head of Justice's civil division said "For far too long, we have heard that the pharmaceutical industry views these settlements merely as *the cost of doing business.*"

GSK pleaded guilty to these crimes of *telling patients their drugs could help when they didn't have evidence of it!*

It is too bad the crime is only a misdemeanor (in Massachusetts), as millions of Americans took Paxil, Wellbutrin, and Avandia *off-label* at the urging of doctors who received "every imaginable form of high priced entertainment, from Hawaiian vacations to millions of dollars to go on speaking tours to a European pheasant hunt to tickets to Madonna concerts, and this is just to name a few," said Carmin M. Ortiz, U.S. attorney in Massachusetts.

And was this some sort of freak event? Some cosmic fluke that was created by a wormhole…?

No.

BUSINESS AS USUAL

This was just the most recent in a string of hundred million/ multi-billion dollar fines paid by the drug companies for illegal practices.

Two months before, Abbot Laboratories pleaded guilty to and paid 1.5 billion for promoting Depakote, a "seizure medication" (more accurately- a drug that has shown SOME improvements in the SYMPTOMS of seizures) for off-label uses. (USA TODAY 5/7/12)

The misconduct was not the product of "some rogue sales representatives," said Heaphy, the U.S. attorney for the western district of Virginia. "The company engaged in the strategy from 1998 to at least 2006"

Depakote is an anti-seizure and mood-stabilizing drug prescribed for bipolar disorder. However, the federal government found that Abbott Labs marketed the drug for unapproved uses, including treatment of schizophrenia, dementia and autism!

In 2009, Pfizer and its subsidiary, Pharmacia & Upjohn, pleaded guilty to a felony violation (in Pennsylvania) for promoting off-label uses of Bextra, such as for pain relief after knee replacement surgery (as well as Lyrica- another "anti-seizure" medication that is now being used for the foot pain associated with diabetic neuropathy.)

They were fined $2.3 Billion (again, with a *B*) *DOLLARS!*

In 2010, AstraZeneca was fined $520 million for this off-label, illegal and dangerous promoting.

The company had "turned patients into guinea pigs in an unsupervised drug test" said U.S. Attorney Michael Levy of Philadelphia, where the settlement was filed.

Partly because of all this *off-label* use of Seroquel, the drug brought in $4.9 billion to the company in 2009 alone, making it the #2 selling drug. (USA TODAY 4/27/10)

And in one of the first and most powerful cases to start off revealing the evil of turning millions of people into guinea pigs for the sake of a profit, in the book Our Daily Meds, Melody Peterson, an investigative journalist included an entire chapter devoted to one of Dr. Russ' favorite medications, Neurontin. (Note: It is hard to write sarcasm onto paper).

Neurontin is the number one drug taken by Dr. Russ' patients for neuropathy. It sometimes helps to numb down the pain, stinging, or burning in many patients who have peripheral neuropathy in their feet.

The problem is: it has never, ever been FDA approved for neuropathy. Yet 90% of his neuropathy patients have tried or are on neurontin (gabapentin) for their neuropathy symptoms.

In fact, like the *other* drugs mentioned previously, it is an "anti-seizure" medication (for certain types of seizures, in addition to other meds). And it is also for a *specific type* of nerve pain called neuralgia- usually as a result of shingles zoster or "herpes outbreak."

Then why are so many patients on this medication- for their foot pain?

Because as Miss Peterson points out in her chapter *"Neurontin for Everything",* Pfizer's marketing machine was pushing doctors to prescribe it illegally: off-labeling it for TONS of different conditions that it was never found to be effective for.

In addition they were pretty much saying "there is no unsafe dose." And the only reason many patients weren't "responders" yet, was that they weren't taking a strong enough dose. So if 300 mg didn't work, just take double! Patients were (and sometimes still ARE when they come into our Neurology office) taking 3,000 milligrams per day!

It was being promoted for migraines, ADHD, bipolar disorder, Restless Leg Syndrome, chronic pain, tremors, Lou Gehrig's disease, and "almost any neurological condition." (p. 223)

... and it still is. (Well, by DOCTORS anyway... who didn't get the memo that it only has two approved uses).

And when a whistle-blower finally came forward, the FDA got wind of it and levied a fine of $430 million dollars.

And this was all the way back in May of 2004.

Patients to this day, are still being told that "Neurontin is for Neuropathy." Only it's not. It's "for seizures." An over-firing brain. So they are getting their brains turned- down, or dulled- down by this inhibitory drug and suffering the numerous side-effects because of some slick marketing by these multi-billion dollar corporations who spend far more each year on marketing than any actual research.

(This directly from Marcia Angell, MD- former editor, New England Journal of Medicine, in <u>The Truth about the Drug Companies</u>).

Some experts estimate that <u>90% of the profits of Neurontin are from the off-label uses! (p. 249)</u>

This is *the* reason why today, patients are being lied to, manipulated, and marketed to aggressively. Because of corporations whose sole purpose is to make their shareholders *money*.

WHAT DOES IT ALL MEAN?

The purpose of all this reading and referencing is this-

The Drug Company's Job is to make its shareholders money by telling you that they can help your health or mood with a pill.

Now, this is at the expense of *actual* science.

In fact, it's easier to avoid science and cheaper (by far) just to hire a celebrity who gives you a good feeling to market a drug for them. (Moynihan/ Cassels 2005) Bob Dole was one of the first pitchmen for Viagra, but Sally Field is still telling us if we don't take her drug, our (grand)mother's bones will turn to ash the moment she hits menopause!

Yet, regarding moods and medication, a large scale review of published research in JAMA (formerly the Journal of the American Medical Association) showed that the "benefit of antidepressant medication compared with placebo increases with severity of depression symptoms and may be *minimal or nonexistent...* in patients with mild or moderate symptoms"! (JAMA 1/6/10)

That's right. if you are feeling a little down and out, the less likely an anti-depressant is to work. Hence, they are saying the evidence is weak that you would feel better if it's mild. It's only if you are suffering from severe depression that it works well.

Yet, the marketing blitz indicates if you are feeling a little low like "Dot," (remember that little Zoloft promotional campaign character? - the bouncing circle?) you should talk to your doctor about taking a drug whose side effects have to take up the last 30 seconds of the commercial! And even then they put silly pictures on the screen to draw your visual attention away from the actual message that should be gotten across to the viewer!

More importantly, current research has shown several important facts:

1. Low vitamin D levels can lower your mood
2. Low Omega 3 levels (EPA and DHA) can, too
3. So can anemia
4. So can a lack of exercise
5. Increased *inflammation* is linked to poorer mental health function
6. Also, the FDA-approved prescribing information for Ambien warns that suicidal thoughts or actions have been reported by depressed patients using this class of drugs (sleep enhancers like zolpidem).
7. Neurofeedback can make lasting changes in patients with everything from anxiety and addiction to depression

But how many of these factors (if any) does the primary care doctor take to address? He's often too busy with cold and flu season. Or seasonal allergy prescriptions about the same time junior needs his Ritalin refill.

All kidding aside. We know that most primary care physicians are very busy and provide very important services for patients with heart disease, infections and life-threatening conditions. But many cases of mood disorders are being treated with "a pill and a pat on the back."

This "rush to prescribe" mentality is at the very core of the problem with our healthcare system in America. It is THE reason most of the drugs prescribed to children for ADHD, depression, or anti-psychotics "involve *off-label* use because efficacy of psychotropic drugs has not been demonstrated in very young children." While methylphenidate "carried a warning against its use in children younger than 6 years." Yet, 1- 1.5% of all children age 2 to 4 years enrolled in Medicaid programs are receiving stimulants, antidepressants, or antipsychotic medications! (JAMA Feb 23, 2000)

These are the reasons to be concerned. These are the exact reasons we are working to help patients get out of the blues and live full and happy lives with children and parents who want to live well!

There are numerous reasons to seek a non-drug approach but we will finish with this point: a growing number of researchers have observed the growing trend of violence and suicidal thoughts associated with mind-altering drugs.

In fact, most of the school shootings, from Columbine to Littleton and beyond have involved shooters who were taking one or more of these anti-depressant, anti-psychotic medications and even ADHD meds.

Since our brain isn't even fully formed in our teen years, we are messing with the very architecture and chemistry that is STILL DEVELOPING when we prescribe these meds to a growing brain.

ANXIETY AND DEPRESSION

A couple months ago, I was going through a lot of family stressors, a lot of anxiety, a lot of depression. [My family doctor prescribed a couple medications for me]. I started with the Neurofeedback and have noticed changes after the first one or two [sessions]. I stopped taking an anxiety medication after the first two. I cut down since we finished 20 sessions, I haven't used ANY anxiety medications. I noticed a LOT of good results with it!

8. SEIZURES, TBI, DEMENTIA, ADDICTIONS, AND OTHER DISORDERS

"Keep an open mind, but not so open that your brains fall out." - Unknown

SEIZURES AND EPILEPSY

Seizures are a condition of over-firing of nerve cells of the central nervous system. They can occur for a multitude of reasons and take many different shapes. A more thorough understanding of what to look for can be seen with a simple Google search. Almost everyone can picture the classic "clonic" portion of a tonic/clonic seizure as the body is "seizing up," shaking uncontrollably or the "tonic" portion when the muscle tone and body tightens/stiffens up.

There are actually numerous other types of seizures that are equally as common. Heather used to have "staring spells" where she would "zone out" but have no memory of the events that passed around her. Her family would just see her sitting there "looking though them." These are classic signs of Absence seizures or even Complex partial seizures if the individual also hallucinates sights, sounds, or smells.

Post-traumatic seizures occur with traumatic brain (head) injuries.

Another common type of seizure is the simple partial where the patient feels weird sensation, twitching or contraction of just a body part. These could include arm, leg or face (grimacing). Another kind, febrile seizures, occur with fevers, but rarely last long .

Note: A seizure is a single event. Epilepsy is having recurrent unprovoked seizures.

Typical treatment for seizures is anti-convulsant medication such as Tegretol or Lamictal mentioned in Heather's story in Chapter one. Other options used frequently are Phenobaritol, Dilantin, Depakote, Neurontin and Lyrica. These are inhibitory chemicals that turn down the brain's function. (They are based on GABA, a neurotransmitter that turns off nerve cells/ inhibits them).

When anti-convulsants do not control the seizures, surgery is often the next step. Brain surgery. Where they cut off a portion of the brain so it can't spread to other areas. Or cut *out* the focal region where the over-firing *begins* and proceeds to spread out from.

For instance if the seizure activity starts in the temporal lobe that spreads to the other lobes on the right side of the brain, they may remove the right temporal lobe. Same if it starts in the parietal lobe and spreads to the frontal or temporal lobes.

They can even put brain-implants in to release medication directly to the brain *or* to discharge an electrical pulse in an attempt to disrupt the over-firing portions (as was recommended to Heather).

If it starts on one side and actually spreads to the other hemisphere, another slightly more invasive procedure is severing the entire corpus callosum, "the bridge" consisting of 200 million nerve fibers that connects the left and right hemispheres of the brain. Patients who agree to this are guaranteed to have split-brain personalities and symptoms. Since the right and left brains can't communicate anymore, the patient *will* develop speech, cognitive, balance and coordination problems (Recall Roger Sperry won the Nobel prize for studying brain regions and split-brain patients).

Not to sound flippant (well, not *too* flippant anyway), but this is basically 1950s medicine practiced *today!* Actually, it's more like *Trepanning*- the Egyptian practice of drilling a whole in the skull to remove the brains before mummification and even for headaches!

Going straight to medication in non-emergency situations is like burning down the barn to get rid of the mice! Numerous other interventions are actually found to help dramatically at bringing the state of the brain back to stable levels. The most basic is diet.

Johns Hopkins reviewed the literature on high fat diet for seizures as being one of the oldest but still misunderstood. Just a decade ago "the ketogenic diet was seen as a last resort; however, it has become more commonly used in academic centers throughout the world even early in the course of epilepsy." (Lancet 2004)

They go on to say "Dietary therapies may become even more valuable in the therapy of epilepsy when the mechanisms underlying their success are understood." Translation: If more doctors were looking at the cause and not just prescribing pills, more people could benefit by just changing their diet!

Other research shows that eliminating certain foods from the diet, like gluten, results in a very favorable outcome. Gluten is a pro-inflammatory protein from wheat. It promotes swelling in the body and brain. (Neurologist. 2006)

Several recent studies are even pointing towards epilepsy as one of the growing list of auto-immune disorders! (Neurology 2005/ Epilepsia 2011) We will discuss more about reducing food triggers via an anti-inflammatory diet in Chapter 9. For now, it's safe to say that a combination of Neurofeedback, high-fat diet, and low-reactive foods (especially to eliminate MSG and its derivatives) are critical aspects to helping seizure disorders.

Heather's story brings to light the importance of addressing the core issues like inflammation in the brain, not drugging for the sake of prescription sales!

CONCUSSIONS/ TRAUMATIC BRAIN INJURIES

A concussion is a type of TBI (Traumatic Brain Injury) caused by a bump, blow or jolt to the head that can change the way your brain normally works. It is often referred to as a "mild" TBI or mTBI.

20-30% will have lingering symptoms that may include:

Difficulty thinking clearly, difficulty concentrating or remembering new information, headache, blurred vision, nausea, vomiting, dizziness, irritability, sadness, and sleep disorders

A history from a family member is often more important because the injury sufferer may not notice these changes themselves.

You should take the victim to the ER immediately if they start falling asleep, have different sized pupils, start convulsing or seizing, start talking nonsense or behave irregularly. Loss of consciousness, as a rule of thumb, needs to be evaluated by a professional.

Concussions and TBIs raise the risk of developing seizures, Alzheimer's disease, Parkinson's and dementia later in life. As mentioned earlier, many pro football players are dying too soon or living too long but forgetting who their own families are *in their 50s!!!* Former quarterback, Jim McMahon of the Chicago Bears is a victim of early onset dementia and helped the players to win the nearly 1 billion dollar lawsuit against the NFL. His fiancé takes regular pictures of him with her so that he doesn't forget who she is.

Studies are showing how impaired eye movements reveal continued post-concussion symptoms. (Brain 2009)

Two recent cases had head injuries over 5 years ago. They also developed nerve damage and burning in their feet. Lots of therapy in the form of functional neurological care helped resolve most of the symptoms. A key was helping to control the ongoing inflammation in the skull itself. Cold laser was important for that alone!

DEMENTIA AND ALZHEIMER'S

"It's hell getting old, but it beats the alternative!"

There is a global crisis coming. It's not here all together yet, but it is growing by the day like a snow-ball rolling slowly downhill at first. It is currently in the process of gaining momentum.

The most recent estimates put the number of sufferers at 44 million worldwide. (The 2010 number was 35 million). By 2030, that number is expected to reach 76 million people. (USA TODAY 12/5/13)

In 35 years, it will be inescapable. By 2050, 135 million people will be living with Dementia (an early form of Alzheimer's disease).

It is being labeled a global epidemic. It is a financial, political and neurological tragedy. There is just no way to support that number of people with healthcare when it happens.

The burden that Alzheimer's and other forms of dementia are poising to place on the world's economies and on the individual families whose loved ones have lost their memories and their ability to function will be catastrophic.

The estimate rose 17% percent when researchers had to account for the number of persons developing symptoms long before age 80! Some are starting to develop in their 60's. A portion in their fifties.

What could account for such an increase? A point that should be made repeatedly is that we don't live in the same environment anymore. Our food supply has been hacked. Our taste buds have been hi-jacked by forms of MSG that didn't exist in the world's food supply until the 1940's.

Dr. Russell Blaylocks book Excitotoxins shows what happens to neurons exposed to high doses of glutamate (in free glutamic acid form) and aspartame. It looks like a tree that has lost it's leaves! It looks dead.

And frankly, that's what IS happening.

Almost all of us are getting these ingredients *daily* through innocent sounding names such as:

Monosodium glutamate (MSG)

Monopotassium glutamate

Anything "hydrolyzed"

Sodium caseinate

Yeast extract

Whey protein

Soy protein

Soy sauce

(see TruthInLabeling.Org for *more* aliases)

Plus, when tested, those with the worst symptoms of dementia/forgetfulness, had the lowest blood concentrations of the Omega 3 *Essential Fatty Acids.* DHA is *the* fatty acid used to grow new synapses, or connections in the brain. And EPA keeps the inflammation down! Talk about a recipe for disaster…

Recent data published in the journal *Neurology* from the Women's Health Initiative Memory Study showed that "higher omega-3 levels may slow the loss of brain volume that occurs as we age." (Neurology 2014)

As of about a decade ago, when researchers discovered that the brain make its own insulin, Alzheimer's was being referred to by the term "Type 3 Diabetes." In many cases, the nerve cells began breaking down and forming the bad (tau) proteins when the brain cells became "numb" to the effects of insulin (called insulin resistance). (Newport 2011) Proper blood sugar levels need to be maintained. Not longer is it acceptable when your doctor says "your not diabetic *yet* but you're a few points away!" Even blood sugar levels barely over 100 can cause nerve damage in the brain or body.

Even adequate vitamin D levels are important for normal brain health. A UK study showed last year that vitamin D deficiency contributes to significant stress in the brain and "may promote cognitive decline in middle-aged and elderly adults." (Free Radical Biology and Medicine 2013)

(Both vitamin D and EPA/DHA blood levels can be tested with a simple blood draw).

So, we all need to do right by our genetics and eat the way we were designed to. (See Chapter 9)

In addition, numerous studies have focused on cold laser for the reduction of inflammation in the brain. Harvard got turned onto this about 5 years ago and has been using lasers on concussion patients and those with neuro-inflammation.

And neurofeedback is now being targeted towards those with neuro-degeneration issues. The idea is that even if some of the nerve cells are dying off, the rest should still be "exercised" (with neurofeedback) as well as cognitive memory games like crossword puzzles and Sudoku. (*J Am Geriatr Soc.* 1/13/14)

Below are actual examples of what starts to happen as the brain deteriorates. While it is known that we are *all* losing brain cells after the age of 25, it is an extremely slow, deliberate process, like losing muscle size.

But what about Jack LaLanne? Had he lost much muscle tone when he died at 96? Was he pretty sharp? It's pretty obvious that he was still as quick as a whip and promoting health through juicing and exercise!

We ALL need to maintain the quality of life of our brains. They have to last us as long as the *rest* of our body!

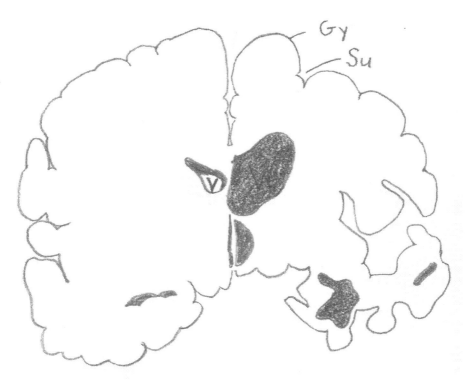

NORMAL   **DEGENERATED**

FIGURE 8.1 Normal vs. Degenerating Brain
Gy= Gyrus, Su= Sulcus, V= Ventricles
This diagram represents a slice of two different brains merged
together. Note the fullness and thickness of the normal brain on the
left. It thoroughly fills up a skull. Contrast that with the severe
atrophy (shrinkage) on the right and the enlargements of the spaces
inside (ventricles= shaded areas). Significant amounts of gray matter
have been lost, contributing to the expansion of the ventricles (fluid-
filled holes inside the brain). The entire temporal lobe can be seen to
almost wither away on the bottom right of the figure.

ADDICTION

Addiction is a disorder that occurs when an individual ingests a substance (alcohol, cocaine, nicotine, sugar/carbohydrates) or engages in an activity (gambling, sex, internet use) that is pleasurable ("feels good"). However, it is the compulsive indulgence in this behavior that causes adverse consequences or interferes with daily responsibilities, work, relationships, or health. Many users are not aware they have a problem.

Here in Ohio, there are multiple southern counties known for marijuana production and crystal meth labs. Marijuana is thought of as being a psychologically addictive drug, as many individuals make a habit out of using it, at the expense of relationships, jobs and positive healthful activities (especially exercise).

Numerous states and doctors are de-criminalizing medical marijuana or "weed" as of 2014 and starting to regulate it like alcohol. Even Dr. Sanjay Gupta, the CNN medical correspondent "Changed His Mind" in a CNN story saying for such conditions as cancer, that the medicinal uses of the active ingredients outweigh the possible side-effects. (8/8/13)

We're not here to judge any specific type of addiction, or the behaviors that result in the first place. But when someone comes to the realization that they have a problem (or when their family does), then it's time to get help.

With the "Meth Labs" growing in popularity, and meth "cookers" dying from explosions that result from improperly handled chemicals, there is a desperate need to reach out to help addicts to overcome their need for a "fix." Families are being destroyed. Children are growing up without parents. Lives are being lost.

Entire criminal ventures are being set up transporting West Virginia addicts or financially destitute individuals by bus down to the pill-mills of Florida for multiple drug prescriptions from multiple establishments. Patients with chronic pain become addicted.

Families lose their incomes. Mothers, fathers, sons and daughters go to jail. It's costly and destroying poorer parts of the country!

But, when you go to PubMed.gov (the National Library of Medicine's research search engine) and type in "Addiction and Neurofeedback," you will come across several current studies where EEG Biofeedback/Neurofeedback was used to help improve mood, reduce cravings and help addictive behaviors.

One study said Neurofeedback has "a substantial body of research... conducted over the past three decades by Peniston using a slow EEG-wave protocol for the treatment of addictive disorders... This "Peniston-Protocol" became very popular and widely accepted... and has shown to be effective in a number of studies." (Frontiers In Psychology 2013)

Neurofeedback has lost its popularity with the development of drugs like Methadone, that reduces withdrawal without causing the "high" associated with the drug itself. Methadone clinics had been popular for addiction-withdrawals, but there is still inherent danger when using prescription drugs anyway.

However, addiction clinics such as Passages Malibu actually use Neurofeedback as one of their protocols to help clients. Some of these clinics can cost around $27,000 for four weeks of care. (PR Newswire 12/7/10)

At Passages Malibu, treatment starts at $64,000 a month! (NY Times 9/13/13)

Neurofeedback is an effective tool for many people. But you shouldn't have to fly to California and spend your car (OR your house) to get the benefits. Neurofeedback, by changing how the neurons in your brain fire, is thought to get its results with addiction by also changing what neuro-chemicals the brain produces.

Other procedures include footbath "detoxes" that pull ionic chemicals out from between the cells. This excess or build-up is believed to be what's left behind when the liver has trouble clearing out the chemicals from the blood.

Dietary intervention is often used since sugar is actually more addictive than cocaine and heroine. (Forbes.com 10/16/2013) This explains why when patients go through such alcohol and drug counseling as Alcoholics Anonymous, that they use 3 other legal drugs: nicotine, caffeine, and jelly donuts.

P.O.T.S. (Postural Orthostatic Tachycardia Syndrome) and Orthostatic Hypotension

Patients with POTS have "racing hearts" that increase by more than 30 beats per minute, to a heart rate exceeding 120 bpm.

Most cases involve relatively young women (14-45 years of age) with a 5 to 1 ratio of women vs. men. The heart races, sometimes even with a drop in blood pressure of 10 to 20 mmHg. (Goldstein 2001)

In Orthostatic Hypotension, a sudden drop in blood pressure usually occurs as the patient rises from a seated to standing position. Because this requires an *increase* in pressure to get blood volume to the head, the lack of blood flow to the brain causes a "fainting spell" or pseudo-seizure that looks as if the patient "staring off into space" while actually unconscious. These resemble and are often mistaken for absence seizures, as well.

A well respected neurologist said to me in 2010, "Every case of POTS I have ever seen has had food issues" – meaning food/gluten sensitivities, excessive inflammation in the brain from diet, and or deficiency of essential fatty acids.

These patients are best benefited with neurological training, dietary restrictions, and supplementation. Neurofeedback may show improvement if a Brain-Map reveals problems. Salt intake is actually encouraged to increase blood volume and therefore blood pressure.

Medical treatment basically consists of drugs that increase blood volume. Patients are encouraged to exercise their calves and wear compression hose on their legs. A simple tip is to bear down like during a bowel movement when you stand up, to support maximal blood pressure.

POST CONCUSSION/ BRAIN-FOG

Three years ago I fell off a horse head first. Since then I'd had this brain-fuzz, and I thought if I'd just shake my head or stomp my feet that it would go away. It was just clouding my thoughts. I've had lots of treatment but nothing has helped... until now! And it has quit! [since coming in to Dr. Russ for 3 months]! I just really noticed that I can think now. It was so bad that I was just ready to give up on life. I'd just sit in a daze. That's how I was all the time! And I couldn't think. I couldn't function. Now I can sit and talk to anybody. I can talk to my husband. My family. I couldn't even talk on the telephone! Now I can!

BEHAVIORAL AND LEARNING CHALLENGES

[In the first month with Dr. Russ and Heather] My son's behavior has *greatly* improved. His ability to catch himself in his anger has increased dramatically. We don't notice as much anger. He struggled in reading and math, but he's got to the point now where another classmate has actually asked to copy off of *his* papers. He's made huge improvements since the start of the school year... It's *harder* math, and he's getting it!

TICS

We met Dr. Russ through some friends at church, and they said he might be able to help our son Tyler with his motor tics. We were so sad for him. Even friends looked at him like he was different because he sounded like he was coughing or clearing his throat several times a minute. We had lost hope in it going away on its own, and the medications never did help much. We took Tyler in to get his nervous system evaluated and Dr. Russ immediately found problems with the firing of some of the nerves in his spinal cord. We started treatments. They were gentle and Ty never complained. After just a couple of months, the constant throat clearing and hacking that he was victim to was practically gone. Dr. Russ also gave him some learning tools to help with words and spelling for school. We just want to thank Dr Russ for helping our son.

TINNITUS/ RINGING IN THE EARS

I had ringing in both ears. I tried everything. I doctored with every doctor who knew anything about it. None of them could help me, so I lived with it. It was constantly the same, constantly ringing and buzzing. I learned to live with it. And that went on for 13 years. I came in about two months ago, and after about the fifth treatment, I began to notice the buzzing was disappearing. Sometimes completely. Which it had never done before. Every trip over here I was hooked up to the machines it got better and better and better and better. And as I sit here today, I don't have one bit of ringing in my head and no buzzing. And I'm sleeping better. My whole life is better. I can hear people's voices clearer. Clear as a bell.

9. NUTRITION AND METABOLISM

"There are a thousand hacking at the branches of evil to
one who is striking at the root."
- Henry David Thoreau

As was noted back in chapter 3 in A Slip On The Ice, the average
American eats a diet loaded in processed foods, Omega 6
(inflammatory) grains, simple sugars, trans fats and MSG
derivatives.

Nutritionists commonly call it the SAD Diet. The Standard
American Diet. Because it's just. plain. sad.

Science changes with the political winds and current opinion.
Remember when there were four food groups. That's what we
learned from Slim Good-body in the 80's (in between episodes of
The Electric Company and Sesame Street).

But a strange thing happened in the late 90's, a strange looking
food *pyramid* began appearing as some nutcases began being
influenced by the grain industry. All of a sudden instead of "just" 4
servings per day of breads and cereals, now we were supposed to get
SIX to ELEVEN!!!

And America's waistlines exploded!

Then about the time of President Obama, a new policy team came into force and the MyPlate paradigm took effect for a new generation of dieters. It knocked the grain servings down to "just" 3 per day and upped the fruits and vegetables to a serving per meal.

Time will tell what the next vision of what "health" looks like on a dinner plate, but countless books from The Crazy Makers to Salt Sugar Fat and The End of Overeating list the numerous SAD statistics of how we are the fattest, sickest persons on the planet-despite the fact that we have been preached at to stay away from fat! (Taubes 2011)

The reality is that we can't trust the cooks in the kitchen of Big Corporations. They are as bad as big tobacco. In fact, Dr. David Kessler was the FDA commissioner back in the 90's who took on big tobacco to expose their lies. He is also author of The End of Overeating, where he exposes the *food* industries manipulation of our taste buds to fool us into craving more of their products at the expense of our health!

More and more books are coming to our rescue about how to get back into balance with our own nutrition. We will not argue the cases that they have made so strongly except to say this-

The world of today is not the same as the one of our great grandparents.

We have toxins, poisons and questionable chemicals in our environment from industry and even in our foods with the permission of big government.

Chemicals are allowed into our food supply UNTIL they are proven to be harmful. Yet a preponderance of evidence shows that chemicals such as the glutamate in mono-sodium glutamate *over*-stimulates nerve cells and leads to damage to appetite control centers in lab rats and diet-cola drinkers (who have consistent weight gain year-after-year *despite* taking in supposedly fewer calories). (Blaylock 1996)

Grains (like wheat, rye, rice, corn and barley) and soy beans are rich in Omega SIX essential fatty acids. These are the inflammatory kinds of fats that lead to the production of Arachidonic acid in the body, which is linked to every degenerative inflammatory process in the body.

Meanwhile our consumption of fish (loaded in ANTI-inflammatory Omega 3s) and vegetables (containing nutrients such as vitamins, minerals and fiber) is lacking... so much so that the U.S. government allowed for the re-labeling of French fries with ketchup to be counted towards the 5 servings of fruits and vegetables recommended on a daily basis.

S. A. D.

It's truly a sad state to see our children turning into extremely obese and unhealthy versions of ourselves as youths. We at least got out of the house to ride bikes. Not only are they phasing out the learning of cursive in school because it is deemed unimportant, many kids aren't even learning to ride bicycles because the parents know they would rather have more time and attention to pay to a new video game!

So please pick up and read some of the works by Mark Sisson or Loren Cordain.

The current favorite that we pre-ordered a week before it even came out is <u>GRAIN BRAIN</u> by David Perlmutter, M.D.

He is a pediatric neurologist who uses a heavy dose of nutrition and life-style changes for his patients with neuro-behavioral disorders. He even explains the role of the immune system in food allergies and sensitivities. In his previous book <u>Raise a Smarter Child by Kindergarten</u>, he proved to be a decade ahead of the popular press in educating doctors and lay people alike on anti-oxidants and "fish oils."

<u>Grain Brain</u> is a complementary follow-up to Dr. William Davis's <u>Wheat Belly</u>. As a Cardio-thoracic surgeon, Davis began investigating the role that inflammatory fats from grains played into the health of millions of Americans taking cholesterol medications. It is a shocking expose into the genetic breeding and modification of strains of wheat designed to be sweeter and tastier than ever before!

Not all experts agree on all individual points. More is being learned each year as research is published and analyzed. The role of the immune system is still being heavily touted as Americans want their cake and to eat it too. ("Doctor, I'm eating gluten-free, dairy-free, and soy-free donuts and ice-cream, but I STILL can't lose weight or clear my head from this funk!")

So, trust me when I tell you that gluten-free is not a fad or life-style, but instead it is Nature's blueprint to eat liberal amounts of meats and vegetables, with a slightly more restricted intake of fruits, nuts, berries and seeds. (A.k.a. Paleo Diet, Primal Diet, Caveman Diet, Garden of Eden Diet)

We may choose our foods, but we don't get to choose our genetics. However, eating lots of natural (and especially organic) foods that are nutrient-rich and calorie-moderate sends information via nutrients into our cells that affects the *expression* of our genes (the field of epigenetics).

So choose natural, organic fresh fruits and vegetables, meat, eggs, nuts and berries to nourish your body instead of filling it with calorie-dense, nutrient-deficient *fake*-foods that many dogs will even turn their noses up at ... until they take their first bite and are HOOKED on the additives the same way we are!

Below is a sample diet plan that has been put together from a collections of works to help manage Gluten sensitivity, Lactose Intolerance, Leaky Gut Syndrome, Diabetes, Hypoglycemia, and even high Cholesterol.

For those with high blood sugar, limit fruit to one serving per day.

For those with seizures, we want to get into a "ketogenic" state as well, so apply the high-blood sugar rule above. (Newport 2011)

Note to those who have a family history, *cancer* cells have abnormal mitochondria (energy producing organelles inside the cells' cytoplasm). Cancer cells thrive in a *sugary*, *acidic* environment. Patients with cancer have a poorer prognosis with high insulin levels. (Nutrition and Metabolism 2011) These individuals would do well to also limit fruit to one or two servings daily but raise the level of vegetables while lowering the amount of protein from meat. (Eggs are acceptable at moderate amounts, however)

More great news, a 2012 government study said healthy food is no more costly than junk food. (USA Today 5/16/12)

WEIGHT LOSS

I've lost 30 lbs in the last 5 weeks on your program! I'm using the [Fat-burning] laser and taking supplements. Everything is pretty simple. The diets not too bad and you can live with it pretty easily and actually you feel better compared to the way I ate before! - 50 year old client

I've lost 24 pounds in just a little over 3 months and I didn't even feel like I was working at it! I haven't added any additional exercise other than what I would normally be getting. - 63 year old client

I came to Zanesville to Dr. Schroder and I've been with him for two months now and I've lost about sixty pounds! - 55 year old client

Last month, I weighed 220. This month I weigh in at 194-195. That means I lost about 25 pounds in four weeks coming here to Dr. Russ! - 57 year old client

(N-SAID) NON-STEROIDAL ANTI-INFLAMMATORY DIET

Foods to eat regularly

When confronted with this nutrition program/ lifestyle/ "diet" many people ask "What CAN I eat?" In fact, you'll be eating the way humans have eaten for most of human history. There's plenty of food that doesn't come from an industrialized farm or a can.

- Most vegetables (except tomato, white potatoes, and corn): asparagus, broccoli, beets, cauliflower, carrots, cucumbers, celery, spinach, lettuce artichokes, garlic, onions, peppers, zucchini, squash, rhubarb, turnips, and watercress, among others.
- Meats: chicken, turkey, fish, beef, pork, eggs, lamb, deer, organ meats, etc. Grass-fed and pastured meats from a local farm and/or organic. Avoid factory-farmed meats that contain antibiotics and hormones. Ask around at your local farm market or go to WestonAPrice.org for quality sources of meat locally .
- Low-glycemic fruits: apricots, apples, peach, pear, plums, cherries and berries, oranges, grapefruit, kiwi, to name a few. [or 1/2 a banana, 7 grapes at a time)
- Coconut: coconut oil, coconut butter, coconut milk, coconut cream, coconut yogurt
- Herbal teas and water- Aim to drink HALF your bodyweight in ounces of water daily (150 lbs = 75 oz. of water per day), Almond milk. Stevia is an acceptable sweetener. Natural spices are good.
- Olives and olive oil. Consume probiotics.
- Nuts and seeds (peanuts are NOT nuts, but legumes/ beans)
- Fermented foods like: sauerkraut, kimchi, pickled ginger, fermented cucumbers, kombucha, water kefir, etc. Avoid the ones with sugars and additives. Enjoy making your own!

Foods to eat sparingly (1-2X per week at most)

- Rice, oats, sweet potatoes, glass of red wine, honey, dark chocolate
- Coffee (only a cup a day if you are addicted, but avoid in general)

Foods to avoid

- ALL sugars and sweeteners, even Agave
- High-glycemic fruits: watermelon, mango, pineapple, raisins, canned fruits, dried fruits, etc.
- Avoid Fruit Juice! (It's mostly sugar.) No pop or cola. No soda.
- Tomatoes and white potatoes
- Grains: wheat, barley, buckwheat, corn, quinoa, etc.
- Dairy: milk, cream, cheese, butter, ice cream, whey, etc.
- Soy: soy beans, soy milk, soy sauce, tofu, tempeh, soy protein, etc.
- Alcohol (see above)
- Lectins—a major promoter of inflammation - found in beans, soy, potatoes, tomato, eggplant, peanut oil, peanut butter and soy oil, among others
- No high-fructose corn syrup, trans fats, no glutamate/MSG, no aspartame, no sodium benzoate
- Processed foods, artificial colors/ flavors/ ingredients
- Canned foods

Utilizing this diet for 3 months straight, you are then free to test out the foods you've avoided. Pick a food category (gluten, dairy, soy, tomatoes, etc) each week to try adding back to your diet. Eat as much as you want for 4 days and see if there are any adverse effects (bowel trouble, headache, itching, breathing difficulties, "heaviness," etc). If you do have any negative effects, please don't continue testing it! Just eliminate that food from your diet plan for at least another year. If you feel fine after 4 days, simply wait another 3 days to start adding *another* class of food in. (This is a classic elimination-provocation diet that has existed for hundreds of years).

Recommended Reading:

Grain Brain by David Perlmutter, MD

The Paleo Diet by Loren Cordain, PhD

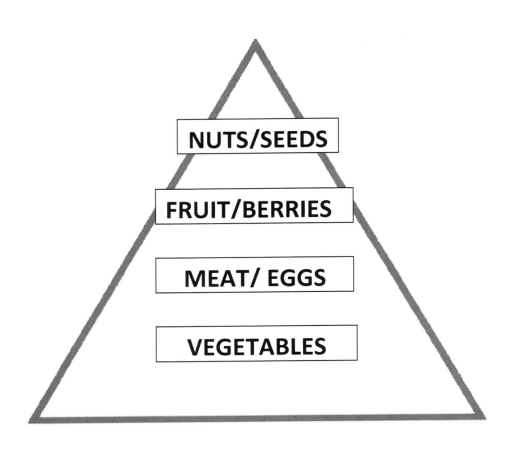

NON-STEROIDAL ANTI-INFLAMMATORY DIET

FOOD PYRAMID

10. QUESTIONS AND ANSWERS

"You can't expect insights, even the big ones, to suddenly make you understand everything. But I figure: Hey, it's a step if they leave you confused in a deeper way."
-    Lily Tomlin, in Jane Wagner's Broadway play,
The Search For Signs of Intelligent Life in the Universe

What Is Neurofeedback?

Our brains can be our best friends or our worst enemy. In 1989, President George HW Bush declared the 90s to be the "Decade of the Brain." Well, in just the past 25 years, we have learned more about how the human brain functions than in _all_ the previous years of recorded human history.

Yet, millions of Americans are suffering. It's a hidden type of suffering that many don't want to share. It makes us feel alone... separated... and empty inside. It is all around us, in our schools and families. We are hurting inside. Anxiety. Depression. OCD. PTSD. Children with behavioral problems that we just can't seem to help without drugging them daily.

Medicine does not have all the answers. It's actually becoming more of a hindrance to those who want to find REAL solutions.

The pill-pushers... Big Pharma. The multi-multi-Billion dollar per year corporations who pay a billion dollars at a time in federal fines for **_breaking the law over and over_** to tell us their "wonder-drugs" will fix every ailment. Abbott. Pfizer. Eli-Lilly. GlaxoSmithKline. The Attorney General said that until we start tossing some of the bosses in jail for breaking laws, then this culture of greed and recklessness will continue. As it is, they just see the billion dollar fines as "marketing expenses" and then go right back to lying about the effectiveness of their drugs (the main law they keep breaking-exaggerated claims and unproven off-label prescription-pushing).

This report will help you to see _how_ to take the drug companies' blinders off for you to see the destruction these pills can cause, to help you get some real answers... real help, so that you or a loved one can eliminate a lifetime of behavioral or emotional disorders and find the peace you desire.

Because, despite having tried your best to cope... you or your child's **behavioral or emotional challenges are constantly getting in the way** of enjoying a good life.

You may be sick and tired of all the drugs and their cost, or are worried about the endless list of side effects which you've read about. We are here to tell you about something scientific, something technological that works with the brain's own natural process of learning and is recognized to help reduce or even ***eliminate the dependence on drugs!***

If you've ever wanted to **explore non-drug, non-surgical alternatives for anxiety, depression, migraines, ADD/ADHD, autism, chronic pain, addiction**, epilepsy and a whole host of other health and behavioral issues, then this may be the most important report you will ever read.

Here at the MIND Institute for Neurological Development...

our goal is to help you to **understand how your brain works, the MIND Institute process**, and the <u>benefits that are possible with</u> **<u>NeuroIntegration</u>**.

Whether you are a mother who is looking to help a child with ADHD or dyslexia, or you have a loved one battling with anxiety, or are even concerned with an emotional/mental problem of your own, you will find the information here easy to read and understand.

Many of our clients, are very intrigued about how Neurofeedback or "EEG biofeedback" works. (Other nicknames include "Brain Biofeedback" or "Neurotherapy" and specifically in OUR office you will routinely hear us say "NeuroIntegration," because our program technically includes the INTEGRATION of *both* Neurofeedback and Audio-visual stimulation... *More on that later.*)

By the time they make it to see us, most clients are **just suppressing the symptoms with the drug regimen** that their doctors prescribed and are becoming **overwhelmed with the increasing cost and side effects of these drugs.**

Our office procedure involves testing a client with a quantitative EEG or "Brain Map", reviewing the initial test results and arriving at a plan of action for reversing the bad wiring in the brain, to help reduce or even eliminate drug dependency by rewiring the brain.

Back in the June 18, 2000 in **Newsweek**, the research authors said -

"The technology is still in its infancy [back in 2000], but its emerging as a tool to treat everything from epilepsy and ADHD to migraines, anxiety, depression, head injuries, sleep disorders and even addiction. In the last few years, neurofeedback has made its way into the offices of hundreds of reputable doctors, psychologists and counselors."

Far more recently, on October 4, 2010, the New York Times extolled the wonders of Neurofeedback and quoted Dr. John Kounis, a psychology professor at Drexel University as saying …

"There's no question that neurofeedback works, that people can change brain activity."

Dr. Russell Barkley, a psychiatrist at the Medical University of South Carolina was highly skeptical at first *until* he was persuaded to look at the latest available research showing **"significant reductions in impulsiveness and inattention."**

Dr. Norman Doidge, MD, psychiatrist and researcher at Columbia University, and author of The Brain That Changes Itself, calls Neurofeedback

"a powerful *stabilizer* of the brain."

He appears regularly on PBS specials describing neuroplasticity- the brains ability to rewire or "learn." [Keep in mind, in 2000 the Nobel Prize in medicine was given to Eric Kandel, PhD for revealing to the world the process of neuroplasticity and ending the dogma of a "hard-wired" brain in adults. Prior to the year 2000, you could even be laughed at in some circles for saying the brain is malleable in adults... Half a century of research and a Nobel prize will certainly put an end to such nonsense as that!]

Dr. Frank Duffy, a professor and pediatric neurologist at Harvard Medical School, and editor of *Clinical Encephalography* stated that -

> **"Neurofeedback should play a major role in many difficult areas. In my opinion, *any pharmaceutical drug that had as wide a range of effectiveness as neurofeedback would be universally accepted and widely used.*"**

Daniel Amen, MD, who also appears regularly on PBS and is the world's leading authority on SPECT scans (hi-tech PET scan imaging) talked about Neurofeedback thoroughly while covering brain technologies in his book <u>Healing ADD</u>. "The patient's brain is hooked up to the computer equipment through electrodes placed on the head." **"The patient is rewarded for producing concentration or beta waves."**

Dr. Amen goes on later to say "A similar treatment to neurofeedback is something called audio-visual stimulation." It was developed at the University of Texas. It is a type of entrainment (or learning) where the brainwaves begin to fire to the rhythms around us. Blinking lights or rhythmical beats fire at specific frequencies and assist in retraining the brainwaves. He lists both as "promising" techniques for treating conditions like ADHD and other concentration or mood problems without medications.

[This is why the term NeuroIntegration applies to OUR unique Neurofeedback program, because it includes this visual component of timed blinking lights.]

In fact, Neurofeedback was discovered **at UCLA in the 1960s** when a research team lead by Dr. Barry Sterman (a neuroscientist) applied EEG leads to the brain of epilepsy patients and found they could *reduce seizures*. Their theory at the time was that because brain cells communicate with each other via a bio-electrical storm of impulses, that by using feedback they could help the patients brain be rewarded for consistent brainwave patterns. The brain could *normalize*, producing both proper electrical signals... *and* proper brain chemistry!

Research has popped up from around the globe. Doing a literature search on the National Library of Medicine's search engine reveals *over 800 papers on "EEG Biofeedback."* They are overwhelmingly positive with a few poorly done studies showing limited to no improvement. (These studies typically didn't include a Brain-Map or "Quantitative EEG" in the first place, which means the treatment wasn't tailored to the patients' specific needs... a hap-hazard approach to treatment if there ever was one! ... THIS is why we do Brain-Maps before ever initiating a Neurofeedback program).

As neurofeedback providers, we've met and helped hundreds of individuals AND families **forced** to deal with the **negative side-effects of drugs** to alleviate the symptoms (but not cure) patients. We frequently cringe when we see our clients' lists of dangerous, expensive and sometimes ineffective drugs that doctors have prescribed. These drugs may be especially hard on young children whose bodies and minds are fragile and still developing.

What is Functional Neurology?

In Functional Neurology we look at the patient as a whole person. Because the brain is not fully developed when we are born, it is our experiences and learnings that develop us into who we are. In essence, this is what drives our nerve pathways to wire up the unique nerve networks in our own brains. If we miss certain developmental milestones or activities, it can set a delay in our wiring. Or if we have injuries to our brains or damage to the nerves themselves, this interferes with normal brain function. Fortunately, with the advent of neuroplasticity, we have come to learn that nerves can grow new connections and strengthen weak areas. (Schroder 2012)

It's all about neuroplasticity- which is the ever-present ability of the nerves in the brain and body to *re*-wire based on the stimuli they receive. It's neuroscience meets classical neurology. It's about the nervous system's networks and pathways that are *supposed* to connect in certain specific ways and how they become injured or fail to develop appropriately.

There are two types of learning, the good kind and the bad kind. When we learn how to run a new computer program, a new grandchild's name, or even a new hobby, that is considered good learning. Neurons in the brain connect with more branches to become effective at a positive task. In cases of chronic pain, the body wires up signals that send *pain* from the body to the brain more efficiently. That is what we call the bad kind of learning.

In our office, we work daily to stimulate the good kind of learning and override or unravel the pain-learning pathways. ADD/ADHD, Dyslexia, Autism, seizures, TBI and other disorders have pathways and networks that either *didn't develop appropriately* or were actually injured). We drive these neurons to build better brains using movement, balance, and the five senses.

114

Functional Neurologists look for these weak or damaged pathways and create rehabilitative strategies to help grow (or re-grow) the deficient networks. (Note: Some nerve networks *over*-fire and need to be calmed).

What is Cold Laser?

Einstein, Lasers, and The Theory of Relativity

You probably remember from science class that Einstein discovered the Theory of Relativity with the mathematical equation $E=mc^2$. Which means "Energy equals Mass times the velocity of *Light* squared". That simply meant that:

Light Is Energy.

It's really that easy. Whether you are feeling the warmth of the summer sun on your skin, staring at a rainbow or just turning on a flashlight, the light that you see or feel is *ENERGY* in the form of photons.

And LASERs are merely *amplified* light sources. (It's what the "L" and the "A" stand for: "Light Amplification.") And if you think that lasers are only used for cutting diamonds or welding NASA's intricate space shuttles together, you're wrong. They can do SO much more!

How does living tissue react to laser light? Good question. Because you wouldn't want the same strength of laser used near your skin as the kind used by the military to shoot down an enemy missile. You can bet on that.

But at the right wavelength and frequency, light in the form of lasers has a positive effect on human and animal tissue. In fact, Jeffrey R. Busford, M.D. at the Mayo Clinic says

"Laser Therapy is really a form of light therapy, and lasers are important in that they are convenient sources of intense light at a

wavelength that *stimulates specific physiological functions."* (1) ["Reference Number 1" at the end]

And Laser Therapy Has Been Used In Europe For Over *30 Years* In The Medical Field!

Australia and Canada are two other countries where medical doctors routinely use cold lasers to treat a multitude of conditions from inflammation and arthritis to circulatory disorders and diabetic ulcers.

They have been using it to treat traumas, inflammation and overuse injuries. It is also used as a successful treatment for pain relief and healing of arthritis conditions.

Now, It's FDA Cleared And Being Used Right Here In The U.S.

The Department of Veteran's Affairs in New York uses cold laser to help heal diabetic ulcers and treat chronic pain in Veterans.

The National Football League uses it to get players back into playing condition week after week.

But what is the biological mechanism of the healing effect of lasers? The University of Wisconsin Medical College found that lasers "stimulate cytochromes in the body that...

increases the energy metabolism of cells.

Cytochromes are part of the 'electron transport chain' that converts sugar into instant energy required by the body to perform all of its activities, such as raising a finger or *healing a wound."* (2)

Real-life translation... cold laser stimulates the metabolism of cells causing them to *heal* or to heal *faster.*

And Lasers reduce inflammation!

When you look at cells exposed to cold laser under a high-powered microscope (And I did last year!) you can actually see the cells move to surround the pin-pointed laser beam. They *love* the light.

It helps the body regenerate cells, reduce inflammation, and promotes an increase in blood supply. At the tissue level, Stanford found that low level (cold) laser treatment even results in increased collagen production. (3)

In Fact: More Than 3,500 Scientific Studies Exist On Cold Laser.

And right now, this very minute, Harvard, MIT, Massachusetts General Hospital in Boston, and The V.A. are using the same laser technology that we have to treat soldiers who are coming back from war with blast-related concussions, TBI, and other neurodegenerative disorders. And they are in the process of large scale studies to reverse the damaging effect of head injuries in football and hockey using cold laser, also.

Stanford university researchers state that **"Lasers are not magical; it is the light that they produce that yields the biological effect. It is the wavelength of light that is important."** (3) Because the wavelength of light is so important, the "Therapeutic Window" is between 600 and 1000 nanometers. Which simply means that for the laser/light therapy to have its therapeutic benefit, the wavelength of the light that it generates must fall within this range.

Our Erchonia lasers emit a 635nm wavelength, which is the most commonly studied because of its ability to knock out inflammation, promote mitochondria growth, and increase ATP's (adenosine tri-phospate - the basic unit of energy in the cell) energy producing effects!

1. *Low Energy Laser Therapy:* Jeffrey R. Busford, M.D., Department of Physical Medicine and Rehabilitation, Mayo Clinic, Rochester, Minnesota

2. *Light Emitting Diodes Aid In Wound Healing*: Henry T. Whelan, M.D., Professor of Neurology, Medical College of Wisconsin

3. *The Photobiological Basis of Low Level Laser Radiation Therapy*: Kendric C. Smith, PhD., Department of Radiation Oncology, Stanford University School of Medicine

What Is The Interactive Metronome?

The Interactive Metronome (IM) is a computer-based analysis and training system that works by measuring an individual's ability to perform a sequence of timed rhythmical claps at various speeds. One or more body parts can be used to create variety or a challenge.

Neurological deficits and weaknesses are measured with the examination. Results are then seen as the system tracks progress with regular repetition. (In simple terms it measures our brain's timing. Its ability to self-regulate).

Overall, it as an assessment tool and therapy that benefits patients by helping communication *within* the brain via coordinated movements. It is used by therapists and other providers for neurological conditions such as:

ADD/ADHD

Dyslexia and Reading Problems

Speech and Language Problems

Autism

TBI/ Concussions

Balance and Coordination Problems

OCD

Cognitive Deficits/Dementia

There exists a growing body of literature describing neural timing (temporal processing) deficits in Neurobehavioral disorders.

To achieve motor learning, we work to encourage patients to complete tasks repetitively and efficiently, thus encouraging higher cognitive processing.

Synchronized timing *within* the brain and *between* the brain and limbs addresses motor skills and feedback from the computer program.

With the MIND Institute's multi-pronged plan (The MIND Method), we are approaching the deficits from neurological, nutritional and technological aspects. This thorough approach leads to some rather exciting outcomes overall.

IM's game-like, audio-visual aspect is very engaging to children and adults alike. It also provides constant feedback at the millisecond level to promote synchronization and timing in the brain.

Exercises can be customized to include a progression of increasingly complex and precisely timed motor movements mixed with gradually higher & faster cognitive processing, attention and decision-making.

Patients who are challenged and can then see measurable improvements are more motivated to continue their training and achieve optimal success.

For instance, many research studies show that children with developmental dyslexia do not perceive auditory timing and rhythm cues in speech as well as other children, leading to learning difficulties with language. Thankfully, research also shows that the right intervention can promote or restore function.

What Is Exercise With Oxygen Therapy?

Exercising while breathing oxygen/ Exercise With Oxygen Therapy (EWOT) effectively increases the amount of oxygen in the blood plasma (the portion of the blood surrounding the cells). This increased oxygen in the plasma can allow the oxygen to be pushed into the body's cells without the aid of the red blood cells. Called the *Law of Mass Action*, it says that if the concentration of a certain compound (example: Oxygen) in a chemical mixture is high enough, chemical combining will take place with *other* elements of the mixture that wouldn't happen otherwise.

Just look at pro-athletes when they are fatigued during a game. Watch a pro-football player who is "gassed" as he heads off to the sideline, takes a seat on the bench and puts the oxygen mask to his face. Then "Boom!" He's ready to go a minute or two later.

And look at how everyone in the hospital with heart, circulation or stroke issues has the nasal cannula (nose tube) resting over their ears but shooting O2 up their nostrils. True, you sure feel 20 years older WHILE you're wearing it, but you begin to get that feeling of energy and the results carry over long after you finish the session!

EWOT technique is very simple. You should wear light, comfortable clothing with EWOT. Depending on your level of fitness, you might begin by exercising on an upper body ergometer (UBE) – "a bicycle for the arms," or on an elliptical or treadmill for 15-30 minutes while breathing 90-95% oxygen from an oxygen concentrator. If you are less conditioned, you may have to work up from 5-10 minutes or by beginning EWOT with vibration instead. (Donatello 2009)

REFERENCES

Authors' Note: While this remains an extensive list of references, it is not exhaustive. We have still chosen only the most pertinent sources to illustrate our points. As this is not a textbook, we chose not to have upwards of 100 references *per chapter* for readability. - R.S. and H.B.

ABC News, Russell Goldman, May 2, 2013

Amen, Daniel Healing ADD 2001

Am J Psychiatry. 1986 Aug;143(8):1004-9. Right-hemisphere deficit syndrome in children. Authors- Voeller KK.

Angell, Marcia The Truth About the Drug Companies: How They Deceive Us and What To Do About It 2004, 2005

Arrowsmith-Young, Barbara The Woman Who Changed Her Brain: And Other Inspiring Stories of Pioneering Brain Transformation 2012

Associated Press November 22, 2013 "More than 1 in 10 kids has ADHD, government survey says"

Blaylock, Russell Excitotoxins: The Taste That Kills 1996

BMC Neuroscience 2009, 10:67 Brain classification reveals the right cerebellum as the best biomarker of dyslexia

Cyril R Pernet*1, Jean Baptiste Poline2, Jean François Demonet3 and Guillaume A Rousselet4

Brain 2009: 132; 2850-2870 Impaired eye movements in post-concussion syndrome indicate suboptimal brain function beyond the influence of depression, malingering or intellectual ability

Brain 2012 Mar;135(Pt 3):935-48. Epub 2012 Feb 10. A tractography study in dyslexia: neuroanatomic correlates of orthographic, phonological and speech processing.

Eaton, Howard Brain School 2011

Cordain, Loren The Paleo Diet: Lose Weight and Get Healthy by Eating the Foods You Were Designed to Eat 2010

Cordain, Loren The Paleo Diet Cookbook: More Than 150 Recipes for Paleo Breakfasts, Lunches, Dinners, Snacks and Beverages 2011

Cordain, Loren The Paleo Answer : 7 Days to Lose Weight, Feel Great, Stay Young 2012

Davis, William Wheat Belly 2011

Demos, J. Getting Started With Neurofeedback 2004

Dev Neuropsychol. 2010;35(6):698-711. Prevalence of neurological soft signs and their neuropsychological correlates in typically developing Chinese children and Chinese children with

ADHD. - Chan RC, McAlonan GM, Yang B, Lin L, Shum D, Manschreck TC.

Doidge, Norman The Brain That Changes Itself: Stories of Personal Triumph from the Frontiers of Brain Science 2007

Donatello, Jeff Energize Your Brain , Change Your Life: An Introduction To Exercise With Oxygen Therapy 2009

Epilepsia. 2011 May;52 Suppl 3:18-22. Autoantibodies and epilepsy.

Evans, J. Handbook of Neurofeedback 2009

Forbes.com "Research Shows Cocaine And Heroin Are Less Addictive Than Oreos" Accessed at:
   http://www.forbes.com/sites/jacobsullum/2013/10/16/research-shows-cocaine-and-heroin-are-less-addictive-than-oreos/

Free Radical Biology and Medicine 2013
   http://www.ncbi.nlm.nih.gov/pubmed/23872023

Frontiers in Psychology . 2013 Oct 1;4:692 EEG-Neurofeedback in psychodynamic treatment of substance dependence. Unterrainer HF, Lewis AJ, Gruzelier JH.

Gastroenterology 2013 - Kirsten Tillisch, Jennifer Labus, Lisa Kilpatrick, Zhiguo Jiang, Jean Stains, Bahar Ebrat, Denis Guyonnet, Sophie Legrain-Raspaud, Beatrice Trotin, Bruce Naliboff, Emeran A. Mayer. Consumption of Fermented Milk Product with Probiotic

Modulates Brain Activity. *Gastroenterology*, 2013; DOI: 10.1053/j.gastro.2013.02.043

Goldstein, David <u>The Autonomic Nervous System in Health and Disease</u> 2001 pp. 526-529

HealthDay News More Kids Taking Antipsychotics for ADHD: Study - *Unapproved uses of these powerful drugs need further investigation, experts say* Tuesday, August 7, 2012

Hyman, Marc <u>The Ultramind Solution</u> 2009

Hyman, Marc <u>Ultraprevention</u> 2003

JAMA - Antidepressant Drug Effects and Depression Severity, January 6, 2010

JAMA- Psychotropic Drug Use in Very Young Children, February 23, 2000

J Am Geriatr Soc. Published online January 13, 2014. Ten-Year Effects of the Advanced Cognitive Training for Independent and Vital Elderly Cognitive Training Trial on Cognition and Everyday Functioning in Older Adults

J Am Acad Child Adolesc Psychiatry. 2009 October ; 48(10): 1014–1022 Widespread Cortical Thinning Is a Robust Anatomical Marker for Attention Deficit / Hyperactivity Disorder (ADHD)

J Learn Disabil. 2000 Jan-Feb;33(1):83-90. Right hemisphere dysfunction in ADHD: visual hemispatial inattention and clinical subtype. Authors- Sandson TA, et al – Harvard Medical

J Pediatr. 2009 May 1;154(5):I-S43. The Emerging Neurobiology of Attention Deficit Hyperactivity Disorder: The Key Role of the Prefrontal Association Cortex. - Authors- Arnsten AF. - YALE Univ, School of Med

J Neurophysiol 90:503-514, 2003. Movements in Attention-Deficit Hyperactivity Altered Control of Visual Fixation and Saccadic Eye Disorder

Kandel, Eric et al. Principles of Neural Science 2013

Kessler, David The End of Overeating: Taking Control of The Insatiable American Appetite 2010

Kharazzian, Datis Why Do I Still Have Thyroid Symptoms? When My Lab Tests Are Normal 2010

Lancet 2002;360:1498-1502, 1507 The Pharmaceutical Industry as Political Player

Lancet 2004;364:823-4 Food colourings and preservatives—allergy and hyperactivity

Lancet Neurol. 2004 Jul;3(7):415-20. More fat and fewer seizures: dietary therapies for epilepsy.

Luria, Aleksandr <u>Higher Cortical Functions In Man</u> 1973

Martin, Jeremy <u>ADHD: Beyond The Meds</u> 2011

Melillo, Robert <u>Autism: The Scientific Truth About Preventing, Diagnosing, and Treating Autism Spectrum Disorders--and What Parents Can Do Now</u> 2012

Melillo, Robert <u>Disconnected Kids</u> 2010

Melillo, Robert, Leisman, Gerry <u>Neuro-Behavioral Disorders of Childhood</u> 2005

Moller, Aage <u>Neural Plasticity and Disorders of The Nervous System</u> 2006

Moss, Michael <u>Salt, Sugar, Fat: How The Food Giants Hooked Us</u> 2013

Moynihan, Ray and Cassels, Alan <u>Selling Sickness: How The World's Biggest Pharmaceutical Companies Are Turning Us All Into Patients</u> 2005

Nakazawa, Ruth <u>The Autoimmune Epidemic</u> 2008

<u>Netter's Concise Neurology</u> – Misulis, K and Head, T 2007

Neurologist. 2006 Nov;12(6):318-21. - Epilepsy and celiac disease: favorable outcome with a gluten-free diet in a patient refractory to antiepileptic drugs.

Neurology. 2003 Nov 25;61(10):1378-85. Foundas, AL et al- Atypical cerebral laterality in adults with persistent developmental stuttering.

Neurology. 2005 Dec 13;65(11):1730-6. Serum antibodies in epilepsy and seizure-associated disorders.

Neurology. 2014;82:435-442. Published online January 22, 2014.

Neuropsychiatry Neuropsychol Behav Neurol. 2000 Apr;13(2):89-100. Right body side performance decrement in congenitally dyslexic children and left body side performance decrement in congenitally hyperactive children. Authors- Braun CM, et al.

Newport, Mary Alzheimer's Disease: What If There Was A Cure? The Story of Ketones 2011

Nutrition and Metabolism, October 2011, 8 (75) Is There a Role for Carbohydrate Restriction in the Treatment and Prevention of Cancer?

PBS *The Secret Life of The Brain*
accessed at: http://www.pbs.org/wnet/brain/episode2/babytalk/

Perlmutter, David Grain Brain 2013

Perlmutter, David Raise a Smarter Child by Kindergarten: Raise IQ by up to 30 points and turn on your child's smart genes 2008

Peterson, Melody Our Daily Meds: How the Pharmaceutical Companies Transformed Themselves Into Slick Marketing Machines and Hooked the Nation on Prescription Drugs 2008

PR Newswire Dec. 7, 2010 - http://www.prnewswire.com/news-releases/passages-malibu-drug-and-alcohol-treatment-center-announces-launch-of-cutting-edge-brain-paint-neurofeedback-therapy-scientifically-proven-to-reduce-addiction-relapse-rate-into-pioneering-holistic-treatment-program-111436514.html
Accessed 1/23/14

Robbins, Jim A Symphony in the Brain: The Evolution of the New Brain Wave Biofeedback 2000

Sacks, Oliver An Anthropologist on Mars 1996

Schroder, Russel Bucket List: Avengers! A Functional Neurologist's Extra Experience In the #3 Movie Of All-Time! 2012

ScienceDaily. from the Annals of Neurology - Autism four times likelier when mother's thyroid is weakened. Retrieved August 15, 2013, from http://www.sciencedaily.com-/releases/2013/08/130813111730.htm

Shaywitz, Sally Overcoming Dyslexia: A New and Complete Science-Based Program for Reading Problems at Any Level 2003

Simontachi, Carol The Crazy Makers: How the Food Industry Is Destroying Our Brains and Harming Our Children 2007

Sisson, Mark The Primal Blueprint: Reprogram your genes for effortless weight loss, vibrant health, and boundless energy 2013

Taubes, Gary Why We Get Fat: And What To Do About It 2011

The Times Recorder, November 10, 2013 "Mental Disorders Rising In Kids" Section 1A

Time Magazine: The Fires Within: Feb. 23, 2004 - Accessed at http://content.time.com/time/magazine/article/0,9171,993419,00.html

USA TODAY - Abbott Labs agrees to pay $1.5 billion over Depakote – Pete Yost 5/7/12

USA TODAY- Estimate: 135 million worldwide with dementia by 2050 – Karen Weintraub 12/5/13

USA TODAY - Healthy food no more costly than junk food, government finds- Nanci Hellmich, 5/16/12

USA TODAY - Immune system may play crucial role in mental health - Karen Weintraub, Special for USA TODAY 12/1/ 2013

USA TODAY- Pfizer fined 2.3 Billion For Illegal Marketing in off-label drug case – Rita Rubin
http://www.usatoday.com/money/industries/health/2009-09-02-pfizer-fine_N.htm

Whitaker, Robert <u>Anatomy of an Epidemic: Magic Bullets, Psychiatric Drugs, and the Astonishing Rise of Mental Illness in America</u> 2010

RESEARCH

Neurofeedback Research

ADHD

Neurofeedback and standard pharmacological intervention in ADHD: a randomized controlled trial with six-month follow-up.

Meisel V, Servera M, Garcia-Banda G, Cardo E, Moreno I.
Biol Psychol. 2013 Sep;94(1):12-21. doi:
10.1016/j.biopsycho.2013.04.015. Epub 2013 May 9.

Significant academic performance improvements were only detected in the Neurofeedback group. Our findings provide new evidence for the efficacy of Neurofeedback, and contribute to enlarge the range of non-pharmacological ADHD intervention choices.

Dyslexia

The effectiveness of neurofeedback training on EEG coherence and neuropsychological functions in children with reading disability.

Nazari MA, Mosanezhad E, Hashemi T, Jahan A.
Clin EEG Neurosci. 2012 Oct;43(4):315-22. doi:
10.1177/1550059412451880.

Neurofeedback training (NFT) is an effective intervention in regulating electroencephalogram (EEG) abnormalities leading to improvements in behavioral deficits, which exist in children with reading disabilities.

The results showed significant improvement in reading and phonological awareness skills.

These significant changes in coherence possibly **indicate integration of sensory and motor areas that explains the improvements in reading skills and phonological awareness.**

<u>Asperger's Syndrome</u>

Neurofeedback outcomes in clients with Asperger's syndrome.

Thompson L, Thompson M, Reid A.
Appl Psychophysiol Biofeedback. 2010 Mar;35(1):63-81. doi:
10.1007/s10484-009-9120-3.

This paper summarizes data from a review of neurofeedback (NFB) training with 150 clients with Asperger's Syndrome (AS) and 9 clients with Autistic Spectrum Disorder (ASD) seen over a 15 year period (1993-2008) in a clinical setting.

Significant improvements were found on measures of attention (T.O.V.A. and IVA), core symptoms (Australian Scale for Asperger's Syndrome, Conners' Global Index, SNAP version of the DSM-IV criteria for ADHD, and the ADD-Q), achievement (Wide Range Achievement Test), and intelligence (Wechsler Intelligence Scales).

The positive outcomes of decreased symptoms of Asperger's and ADHD (including a decrease in difficulties with attention, anxiety, aprosodias, and social functioning) plus improved academic and intellectual functioning, provide preliminary support for the use of neurofeedback as a helpful component of effective intervention in people with AS.

Autism

The relative efficacy of connectivity guided and symptom based EEG biofeedback for autistic disorders.

Coben R, Myers TE.

Appl Psychophysiol Biofeedback. 2010 Mar;35(1):13-23. doi: 10.1007/s10484-009-9102-5. Epub 2009 Aug 1.

Different patterns of hyper- and hypo-connectivity have been identified with the use of quantitative electroencephalography (QEEG), which may be amenable to neurofeedback. In this study, we compared the results of two published controlled studies examining the efficacy of neurofeedback in the treatment of autism.

Although both methods demonstrated significant improvement in symptoms of autism, connectivity guided neurofeedback demonstrated greater reduction on various subscales of the Autism Treatment Evaluation Checklist (ATEC).

Our findings suggest that an approach guided by QEEG based connectivity assessment may be more efficacious in the treatment of autism.

Autism Spectrum

Neurofeedback for autistic spectrum disorder: a review of the literature.

Coben R, Linden M, Myers TE.

Appl Psychophysiol Biofeedback. 2010 Mar;35(1):83-105. doi: 10.1007/s10484-009-9117-y.

Neurofeedback is a noninvasive approach shown to enhance neuroregulation and metabolic function in ASD.

Dementia/Mild Cognitive Impairment

Quantitative EEG in progressing vs stable mild cognitive impairment (MCI): results of a 1-year follow-up study.

Authors
Luckhaus C, et al.
Int J Geriatr Psychiatry. 2008 Nov;23(11):1148-55. doi: 10.1002/gps.2042.

OBJECTIVE: **The study objective is to evaluate the use of qEEG data for the cross-sectional differentiation of mild cognitive impairment (MCI) from mild Alzheimer's disease (AD) and in the longitudinal prediction of cognitive decline in MCI.**

CONCLUSIONS: **qEEG revealed decreased alpha activity in progressing MCI and mild AD prior to an increase of slow wave activity, which typically occurs in advancing AD.**

Tinnitus/Ringing in the ears

Neurofeedback for treating tinnitus.

Dohrmann K, Weisz N, Schlee W, Hartmann T, Elbert T.
Prog Brain Res. 2007;166:473-85.

Many individuals with tinnitus have abnormal oscillatory brain activity.

Participants who successfully modified their oscillatory pattern profited from the treatment to the extent that the tinnitus sensation became completely abolished. Overall, this neurofeedback training was significantly superior in reducing tinnitus-related distress than frequency discrimination training.

Anxiety

Orbitofrontal cortex neurofeedback produces lasting changes in contamination anxiety and resting-state connectivity.
Scheinost D, Stoica T, Saksa J, Papademetris X, Constable RT, Pittenger C, Hampson M.
Transl Psychiatry. 2013 Apr 30;3:e250. doi: 10.1038/tp.2013.24.

Department of Biomedical Engineering, Yale University, New Haven, CT, USA.
Abstract

We observed changes in connectivity several days after the completion of NF training, demonstrating that such training can lead to lasting modifications of brain functional architecture.

Changes in resting-state connectivity in the target orbitofrontal region **correlated with these improvements in anxiety. Matched subjects undergoing a sham feedback control task showed neither a reorganization of resting-state functional connectivity nor an improvement in anxiety.** These data suggest that **NF can enable enhanced control over anxiety** by persistently reorganizing relevant brain networks and thus support the potential of NF as a clinically useful therapy.

Depression

EEG-based upper-alpha neurofeedback for cognitive enhancement in major depressive disorder: A preliminary, uncontrolled study.

Escolano C, Navarro-Gil M, Garcia-Campayo J, Minguez J.

Conf Proc IEEE Eng Med Biol Soc. 2013;2013:6293-6. doi: 10.1109/EMBC.2013.6610992.

Abstract

The behavioral results showed the effectiveness of this intervention in a variety of cognitive functions such as working memory, attention, and executive functions.

Addiction

Neurofeedback training for opiate addiction: improvement of mental health and craving.

Dehghani-Arani F, Rostami R, Nadali H.
Appl Psychophysiol Biofeedback. 2013 Jun;38(2):133-41. doi: 10.1007/s10484-013-9218-5.

Psychological improvements in patients with substance use disorders have been reported after neurofeedback treatment. However, neurofeedback has not been commonly accepted as a treatment for substance dependence. This study was carried out to examine the effectiveness of this therapeutic method for opiate dependence disorder.

The study supports the effectiveness of neurofeedback training as a therapeutic method in opiate dependence disorder, in supplement to pharmacotherapy.

Functional Neurology Research

<u>ADHD</u>

Brain gray matter deficits at 33-year follow-up in adults with attention-deficit/hyperactivity disorder established in childhood.

Authors

Proal E, et al.

Journal

Arch Gen Psychiatry. 2011 Nov;68(11):1122-34.

Abstract

OBJECTIVES: To test whether adults with combined-type childhood ADHD exhibit cortical thinning and decreased gray matter in regions hypothesized to be related to ADHD and to test whether anatomic differences are associated with a current ADHD diagnosis, including persistent vs remitting ADHD.

DESIGN: Cross-sectional analysis embedded in a 33-year prospective follow-up at a mean age of 41.2 years.

CONCLUSIONS: **Anatomic gray matter reductions are observable in adults with childhood ADHD**, regardless of the current diagnosis.

Exploratory analyses suggest that **diagnostic remission may result from compensatory maturation of prefrontal, cerebellar, and thalamic circuitry.**

Reversing Pathology with Neuroplasticity

Reversing pathological neural activity using targeted plasticity

Nature. 2011 February 3; 470(7332): 101–104.
doi:10.1038/nature09656.

Navzer D. Engineer[1,2], **Jonathan R. Riley**[1], **Jonathan D. Seale**[1], **Will A. Vrana**[1], **Jai A. Shetake**[1], **Sindhu P. Sudangunta**[1], **Michael S. Borland**[1], and **Michael P. Kilgard**[1]

Abstract

Brain changes in response to nerve damage or cochlear trauma can generate pathological neural activity that is believed to be responsible for many types of chronic pain and tinnitus[1–3]. Several studies have reported that the severity of chronic pain and tinnitus is correlated with the degree of map reorganization in somatosensory and auditory cortex, respectively[1,4]. Direct electrical or transcranial magnetic stimulation of sensory cortex can temporarily disrupt these phantom sensations[5].

Repeatedly pairing tones with brief pulses of vagus nerve stimulation completely eliminated the physiological and behavioural correlates of tinnitus in noise-exposed rats. These improvements persisted for weeks after the end of therapy. This method for restoring neural activity to normal may be applicable to a variety of neurological disorders.

Brain Degeneration

Decrease of thalamic gray matter following limb amputation.

Draganski B, Moser T, Lummel N, Gänssbauer S, Bogdahn U, Haas F, May A.

Neuroimage. 2006 Jul 1;31(3):951-7. Epub 2006 Mar 7.

Source

Department of Neurology, University of Regensburg, Germany.

Abstract

Modern neuroscience has elucidated general mechanisms underlying the functional plasticity of the adult mammalian brain after limb deafferentation.

Subjects with limb amputation exhibited a decrease in gray matter of the posterolateral thalamus contralateral to the side of the amputation.

Phantom limb pain was unrelated to thalamic structural variations, but was positively correlated to a decrease in brain areas related to the processing of pain.

The unilateral thalamic differences may reflect a structural correlate of the loss of afferent input as a secondary change following deafferentation.

Brain Degeneration

Central nervous system reorganization in a variety of chronic pain states: a review.

Henry DE, Chiodo AE, Yang W.

PM R. 2011 Dec;3(12):1116-25. doi: 10.1016/j.pmrj.2011.05.018.

Department of Developmental and Rehabilitative Pediatrics, Children's Hospital, Cleveland Clinic, Cleveland, OH 44104, USA. henryd@ccf.org

Abstract

It is now clear that substantial functional and structural changes, or plasticity, in the central nervous system (CNS) are associated with many chronic pain syndromes.

Changes in the motor and sensory homunculus also are seen. Some of these CNS changes return to a normal state with resolution of the pain. It is hoped that this knowledge will lead to more effective treatments or even new preventative measures.

These clinical entities include nonspecific low back pain, fibromyalgia, complex regional pain syndrome, postamputation phantom pain, and chronic pain after spinal cord injury.

Brain Degeneration

Brain Gray Matter Decrease In Chronic Pain Is The Consequence and Not The Cause of Pain

Rea Rodriguez-Racke, Andreas Niemeier, Wolfgang Ruether, and Arne May

The Journal of Neuroscience, November 4 , 2009- 29(44):13746-13750

Abstract

As gray matter decrease is at least partly reversible when pain is successfully treated, we suggest that the gray matter abnormalities in chronic pain do not reflect brain damage but rather are a reversible consequence of chronic nociceptive transmission, which normalizes when the pain is adequately treated.

Cold Laser (LLLT) Research

Neurodegeneration

Low-level laser therapy regulates microglial function through Src-mediated signaling pathways: implications for neurodegenerative diseases.

Song S, Zhou F, Chen WR.

Author information

Abstract

BACKGROUND:

Activated microglial cells are an important pathological component in brains of patients with neurodegenerative diseases.

CONCLUSIONS:

The present study underlines the importance of Src in suppressing inflammation and enhancing microglial phagocytic function in activated microglia during LLLT stimulation. **We have identified a new and important neuroprotective signaling pathway that consists of regulation of microglial phagocytosis and inflammation under LLLT treatment. Our research may provide a feasible therapeutic approach to control the progression of neurodegenerative diseases.**

TBI, stroke, spinal cord injury, and degenerative central nervous system diseases.

The Nuts and Bolts of Low-level Laser (Light) Therapy

Hoon Chung[1,2], Tianhong Dai[1,2], Sulbha K. Sharma[1], Ying-Ying Huang[1,2,3], James D. Carroll[4], and Michael R. Hamblin[1,2,5]

[1]Wellman Center for Photomedicine, Massachusetts General Hospital, Boston, MA, USA
[2]Department of Dermatology, Harvard Medical School, Boston, MA, USA
[3]Aesthetic and Plastic Center of Guangxi Medical University, Nanning, People's Republic of China
[4]Thor Photomedicine Ltd, 18A East Street, Chesham HP5 1HQ, UK
[5]Harvard-MIT Division of Health Sciences and Technology, Cambridge, MA, USA

Abstract
Soon after the discovery of lasers in the 1960s it was realized that laser therapy had the potential to improve wound healing and reduce pain, inflammation and swelling. In recent years the field sometimes known as photobiomodulation has broadened to include light-emitting diodes and other light sources, and the range of wavelengths used now includes many in the red and near infrared. The term "low level laser therapy" or LLLT has become widely recognized and implies the existence of the biphasic dose response or the Arndt-Schulz curve. This review will cover the mechanisms of action of LLLT at a cellular and at a tissular level and will summarize the various light sources and principles of dosimetry that are employed in clinical practice. **The range of diseases, injuries, and conditions that can be benefited by LLLT will be summarized with an emphasis on those that have reported randomized controlled clinical trials.** Serious life-threatening diseases such as stroke, heart attack, spinal cord injury, and traumatic brain injury may soon be amenable to LLLT therapy.

LLLT is also being considered as a viable treatment for serious neurological conditions such as traumatic brain injury (TBI), stroke, spinal cord injury, and degenerative central nervous system disease.

Inflammation of Brain and Nerves

Neurological and psychological applications of transcranial lasers and LEDs.

Rojas JC, Gonzalez-Lima F.

Biochem Pharmacol. 2013 Aug 15;86(4):447-57. doi: 10.1016/j.bcp.2013.06.012. Epub 2013 Jun 24.

Author information

Abstract

Transcranial brain stimulation with low-level light/laser therapy (LLLT) is the use of directional low-power and high-fluency monochromatic or quasimonochromatic light from lasers or LEDs in the red-to-near-infrared wavelengths to modulate a neurobiological function or induce a neurotherapeutic effect in a nondestructive and non-thermal manner.

LLLT is a potential non-invasive treatment for cognitive impairment and other deficits associated with chronic neurological conditions, such as large vessel and lacunar hypoperfusion or neurodegeneration. Brain photobiomodulation with LLLT is paralleled by pharmacological effects of low-dose USP methylene blue, a non-photic electron donor with the ability to stimulate cytochrome oxidase activity, redox and free radical processes. **Both interventions provide neuroprotection and cognitive enhancement by facilitating mitochondrial respiration**, with hormetic dose-response effects and brain region activational specificity.

Alzheimer's Disease

Low level laser therapy rescues dendrite atrophy via upregulating BDNF expression: implications for Alzheimer's disease.

Meng C, He Z, Xing D.

J Neurosci. 2013 Aug 14;33(33):13505-17. doi: 10.1523/JNEUROSCI.0918-13.2013.

Source

MOE Key Laboratory of Laser Life Science and Institute of Laser Life Science, College of Biophotonics, South China Normal University, Guangzhou 510631, China.

Abstract

Downregulation of brain-derived neurotrophic factor (BDNF) in the hippocampus occurs early in the progression of Alzheimer's disease (AD). Since **BDNF plays a critical role in neuronal survival and dendrite growth**, BDNF upregulation may contribute to rescue dendrite atrophy and cell loss in AD. Low-level laser therapy (LLLT) has been demonstrated to regulate neuronal function both in vitro and in vivo. In the present study, **we found that LLLT rescued neurons loss and dendritic atrophy via upregulation of BDNF** in both Aβ-treated hippocampal neurons and cultured APP/PS1 mouse hippocampal neurons.

Together, these studies suggest that upregulation of BDNF with LLLT by activation of ERK/CREB pathway **can ameliorate Aβ-induced neurons loss and dendritic atrophy, thus identifying a novel pathway by which LLLT protects against Aβ-induced neurotoxicity**. Our research may provide a feasible therapeutic approach to control the progression of AD.

Interactive Metronome Research

Dyslexia/Reading Impairment

Reading Intervention Using Interactive Metronome in Children With Language and Reading Impairment

A Preliminary Investigation

1. Michaela Ritter, EdD1
2. Karen A. Colson, PhD1
3. Jungjun Park1

1. *1Baylor University, Waco, TX, USA*

1. Michaela Ritter, Baylor University, One Bear Place, 1300 S. 7th, Waco, TX 76798, USA Email: Michaela_Ritter@baylor.edu

Abstract

This exploratory study examined the effects of Interactive Metronome (IM) when integrated with a traditional language and reading intervention on reading achievement. during a four-week period. **Although both groups made gains in reading rate/fluency and comprehension, the extent of the gains was much larger in the IM group.** IM training may be useful for promoting the reading rate/fluency and comprehension of children with language and reading impairments.

ADHD

Effects of motor sequence training on attentional performance in ADHD children

Gerry Leisman 1,2, * and Robert Melillo 1,3
1 FR Carrick Institute for Clinical Ergonomics , Rehabilitation and Applied Neuroscience, Garden City,

NY , USA
2 University of Haifa , Mt Carmel, Haifa , Israel
3 Department of Psychology , DeMontfort University,
Leicester , UK

Abstract

In this paper we will examine how IM affects human cognitive and neuromotor capacities and functioning and how signal detection methods may be used to functionally evaluate treatment efficacy as well as identifying clinical populations and characteristics for rhythmic training is likely to have a positive effect.

Rhythm feedback training appears to have a significant effect on clinically observed changes in behavior in attention deficit/hyperactivity disorder (ADHD) elementary school-age children.

Effect of interactive metronome training on children with ADHD.

Shaffer RJ, Jacokes LE, Cassily JF, Greenspan SI, Tuchman RF, Stemmer PJ Jr.

Abstract Am J Occup Ther. 2001 Mar-Apr;55(2):155-62.

RESULTS:

A significant pattern of improvement across 53 of 58 variables favoring the **Interactive Metronome** treatment was found. Additionally, several significant differences were found among the treatment groups and between pretreatment and posttreatment factors on performance in areas of attention, motor control, language processing, reading, and parental reports of improvements in regulation of aggressive behavior.

CONCLUSION:

The **Interactive Metronome** training appears to facilitate a number of capacities, including attention, motor control, and selected academic skills, in boys with ADHD.

TBI

Effects of Interactive Metronome Therapy on Cognitive Functioning After Blast-Related Brain Injury: A Randomized Controlled Pilot Trial

Lonnie A. Nelson, Margaret MacDonald, Christina Stall, and Renee Pazdan
Defense and Veterans Brain Injury Center, Fort Carson, Colorado

Objective: We report preliminary findings on the efficacy of interactive metronome (IM) therapy for the remediation of cognitive difficulties in soldiers with persisting cognitive complaints following blast related mild-to-moderate traumatic brain injury (TBI).
 Results: Significant group differences (SRC vs. IM) were observed for RBANS Attention (p _ .044), Immediate Memory (p _ .019), and Delayed Memory (p _ .031) indices in unadjusted analyses, **with the IM group showing significantly greater improvement** at Time 2 than the SRC group, with effect sizes in the medium-to-large range in the adjusted analyses for each outcome (Cohen's d _ 0.511, 0.768, and 0.527, respectively). Though not all were statistically significant, effects in **21 of 26 cognitive outcome measures were consistently in favor of the IM treatment group**

Conclusion: **The addition of IM therapy to SRC appears to have a positive effect on neuropsychological outcomes for soldiers who have sustained mild-to-moderate TBI and have persistent cognitive complaints after the period for expected recovery has passed.**

Oxygen Research

Headaches

JAMA (Journal of the American Medical Association) December 9, 2009

Anna S. Cohen, Ph.D., (National Hospital for Neurology and Neurosurgery, London) and colleagues conducted a randomized, placebo-controlled trial of high-flow oxygen for patients suffering with cluster headaches.

Researcher found 78 percent of the patients receiving oxygen reported being pain-free or have adequate relief within **15 minutes** of treatment, compared to 20 percent of patients who received standard atmospheric air in the room. At 30 minutes and even at 60 minutes, treatment with oxygen was superior to air. There were no serious adverse events from the oxygen.

"To our knowledge, this is the first adequately powered trial of high-flow oxygen compared with placebo, and it confirms clinical experience and current guidelines that inhaled oxygen can be used as an acute attack therapy for episodic and chronic cluster headache,"

Nerve Pain

Hyperbaric Oxygenation Therapy Alleviates Chronic Constrictive Injury–Induced Neuropathic Pain and Reduces Tumor Necrosis Factor-Alpha Production

Fenghua Li, MD,* Lili Fang, MD,* Shiwei Huang, MD,* Zhongjin Yang, MD,* Jyotirmoy Nandi, PhD,*
Sebastian Thomas, MD,† Chung Chen, PhD,‡ and Enrico Camporesi, MD§

(Anesth Analg 2011;113:626–33)

CONCLUSION: These data show that **HBOT alleviates CCI-induced neuropathic pain and inhibits endoneuronal TNF- alpha production,** but not IL-1 in CCI-induced neuropathic pain. Reduced TNF-alpha production may, at least in part, contribute to the beneficial effect of HBOT.

Brain Activation/Verbal Cognitive Performance

The effect of transient increase in oxygen level on brain activation and verbal performance

Soon-Cheol Chunga, Jin-Hun Sohnb, , , Bongsoo Leea, Gye-Rae Tacka, Jeong-Han Yia, Ji-Hye Youa, Jae-Hun Juna and Richard Sparacioc
aDepartment of Biomedical Engineering, Konkuk University, South Korea
bDepartment of Psychology, Chungnam National University, Daejeon, 305-764, South Korea cArmy Substance Abuse Program, US Army, South Korea

Received 27 August 2005; revised 9 February 2006; accepted 23 February 2006. Available online 6 May 2006.

Abstract
This study aimed to investigate the hypothesis that a transient increase in oxygen level administered to subjects increases the BOLD effect in brain regions associated with verbal cognitive functioning and enhances performance accuracy

The neural activations were observed at the occipital, parietal, temporal and frontal lobes, during both 21% and 30% oxygen administration. Increased brain activations were with 30% oxygen administration.

These results suggest **that a higher concentration of breathed oxygen increases saturation of blood oxygen in the brain, and facilitates verbal cognitive performance.**

Proud Members of The:

Pastoral Medical Association

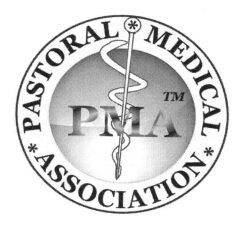

Because more and more families are realizing the importance of safe natural health care options and they want to be sure their provider is a qualified professional.

Because network members have access to a professional level of natural options, self care education and professional advice and assistance right in their own hometown.

www.PMAi.us

Protecting YOUR health care freedoms.

RESOURCES

NEURO CARE/ MIND Institute for Neurological Development

MindOhio.com

OhioAdhdDoc.com

740-588-3339

D-C Chiropractic Neurology Center (main site)

AskDrRuss.com

740-454-1747

American College of Functional Neurology

acfnsite.org

American Chiropractic Neurology Board

acnb.org

The Carrick Institute

CarrickInstitute.org

Interactive Metronome

InteractiveMetronome.com

The Neuro-Metabolic Super Group (Over 300 Functional Medicine Doctors consulted with since 2009)

LifeChangingCare.com

ABOUT THE AUTHORS

Dr. Heather Schroder (formerly Bennett) spent much of her life traveling to doctors and hospitals for documented conditions, some starting at birth. Her medical records consist of numerous doctors' files, each over an inch thick: from her very first stay in the hospital with jaundice as a premature baby, through being diagnosed with "SJS"/ Stevens-Johnson Syndrome (a "one in a million" adverse reaction to her seizure medication that caused much of her hair and skin to fall off), to a diagnosed "heart condition" (involving the nerves to the heart mis-firing) called P.O.T.S. in which the cardiologist was recommending a pace-maker (at age 35!). Throughout all of this, she developed IBS, eczema and clinical depression.

This all changed after a chance encounter with Dr. Russ Schroder, who utilized basic neurological and nutritional principles to give her back her life! Now, working together at Neuro Care, they integrate these techniques and technology to help others regain their lives, as well.

She has an Associates degree in Early Childhood Development, spending a decade working with pre-schoolers and developmentally-delayed children. She left to begin a dance studio while spending 3 years in social work, helping at-risk infants and toddlers as well as adolescents with mental health issues. She has received extensive training in Neurofeedback and the Interactive Metronome and served as the Director of Neuro Care (formerly the MIND Institute for Neurological Development) since 2012. She received her Naturopath Degree in 2017.

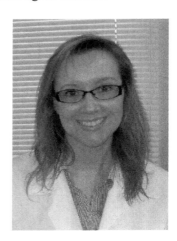

Dr. Heather Schroder, ND – Doctor of Naturopathy

Dr. Russ Schroder graduated with Honors, receiving Bachelors of Science and Doctor of Chiropractic degrees from Palmer College in 1999.

In 2011, he completed a 3-year post-doctoral neurology program through the Carrick Institute for Graduate Studies, successfully passing the 4-day examinations leading to the certification of *Diplomate* of the American Chiropractic Neurology Board and *Fellow* in the American College of Functional Neurology. He is a national lecturer and Charter Member of the International Association of Functional Neurology and Rehabilitation who has expanded the D-C Chiropractic Neurology Center to assist in the non-drug care of patients with chronic pain disorders (such as Peripheral Neuropathy, Degenerative Disc Disease and Fibromyalgia) and metabolic disorders (ranging from thyroid problems to Diabetes). At the M.I.N.D. Institute for Neurological Development, he works with children and adults suffering from Neuro-developmental disorders (such as ADHD, Autism Spectrum Disorders, Learning disorders and Traumatic Brain Injuries). He was certified as a Diplomat in Pastoral Science in 2012 and a Doctor of Pastoral Medicine in 2013 by the Pastoral Medical Association.

He resides in Zanesville, Ohio, focusing on improving the lives of patients with disabling neurological disorders using Functional Neurology, Nutrition and Cold Laser-Decompression. His patients commute from throughout Ohio and its surrounding states to receive his unique and specialized care. His first book *Bucket List: Avengers! A Functional Neurologist's Extra Experience in the #3 Movie of All-Time!* is available on amazon.com

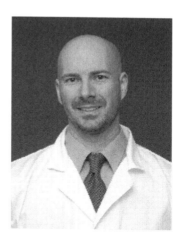

Dr. Russ Schroder, DC, BS, DACNB, FACFN, DPSc, DM (P)

Made in the USA
Lexington, KY
28 May 2018